I Almost Feel Thin

Albert J. Stunkard, M.D.

Bull Publishing Co.

Cover design: Tonya Carpenter
Interior design: Jill Casty

© Copyright 1977
Bull Publishing Co.
P.O. Box 208
Palo Alto, California 94302

ISBN 0-915950-11-1
Library of Congress
Catalog No. 77-70403

contents

Introduction

This is a book about troubled people—those troubled by the modern American obsession with overweight and obesity. It tells something about the way they eat, how they feel about themselves and their bodies, and a good bit about how they cope with the preoccupation that dominates their lives: losing weight.

It tells this tale from a special, privileged vantage point, that of the clinical investigator. There hasn't been a great deal of popular writing about clinical investigators lately. Years ago Sinclair Lewis told us about *Arrowsmith,* and Paul de Kruif about *Microbe Hunters.* But nowadays we read about either clinicians or investigators, not about people filling both roles in their work.

James Watson's *The Double Helix* told a spell-binding tale about how the structure of DNA was deciphered, and several popular medical books have contained moving accounts of people in the throes of physical and mental illness. But the research in *The Double Helix* was not concerned with patients, and popular medical writing has rarely described how the care of patients can advance our understanding of health and disease.

It is as if there were an unbridgeable chasm between medical research and patient care. Yet in reality that chasm has been bridged, and the clinical investigators who have bridged it are responsible for many of the advances of modern medicine.

Theirs is a fascinating story: Part physician, part scientist, the clinical investigator has been given the precious opportunity of caring for patients, and in numbers small enough to permit systematic inquiry into the nature of their problems.

When I first came to psychiatry, there were very few clinical investigators, and very little investigation of any kind. The field was a crude, empirical discipline, very much like the internal medicine and surgery of a hundred years ago. We cared for disturbed and unhappy patients in a manner handed down by custom. We had no specific treatments for the vast majority of patients who came or were brought to us, and no idea of how to go about devising such treatments. Now, in one professional lifetime, all this has changed. The development of research is giving psychiatry a scientific base.

This book deals with some early, uncertain steps in the development of psychiatric research. They were typical of the handful of young research psychiatrists who were attempting to bring orderly methods of investigation to the inchoate field of human behavior and emotions.

Like the others, I had been strongly influenced by psychoanalysis, then the dominant theory in the field. For a time psychoanalysis had made it seem as if a new and fundamental understanding of the human condition was at hand—not just the relief of symptoms but the very transformation of human nature itself. But the bold and far-reaching theories which had stirred the enthusiasm of a generation of psychiatrists seemed unable to generate a systematic program of research. And as theory succeeded theory we seemed as far as ever from a body of cumulative science which is progressively refined by new observations and experiments.

These experiences led some of us to avoid the preoccupation with theory which had so beguiled our teachers, and to look instead toward more prosaic and tangible problems. We tried to describe our patients and what they did just as precisely and with as few preconceptions as we could. And we took special pains in formulating the questions which we asked—to assure that they be at least potentially answerable by our research. The old global inquiries into love and hate were replaced by more modest ones. For me, in my research in obesity, this meant turning away from questions about the *meaning* of overeating and obesity, to more objectively observable issues: Did obese people have special ways of eating? How did their social background and their physical activity affect their weight? How did they feel about being fat?

For years I pursued this research with little hope of seeing the day when we would move beyond our cumbersome and too-often ineffectual methods of treating the obese. It seemed for a long time as if the most that we could look forward to was a slow increase in understanding; we clung to the belief that one day, our work would make a difference. And now it seems as if that time may be approaching. From a variety of fields come signals that help is on the way. New medications, new surgical treatments, and new diets all portend a better day for overweight people. And in psychology the steady progress of behavior modification has brought new hope. But that is getting ahead of the story.

While writing this book I have thought of those who I hope will read it. First, are the large number of overweight and obese people to whom these efforts have as yet brought so little comfort. They should at least know how we have tried. Second, are their friends and relatives. If not already aware, they should understand the pain of obesity. Third, are all those students considering medical research, who may have little idea of the intensely personal experiences behind the limited, tidy perfection of research reports. For some, this account should be encouraging. Others may find the disorder too much to contemplate, and may welcome the early warning.

Finally, I have been writing to everyone whose taxes have supported this work. This book is an accounting to the American people. For a time government support of medical research increased rapidly. Now it is not increasing, and may even be declining. In either case the taxpayers have had very little to say about the matter. Perhaps this account will help them be better informed about the subject, and less vulnerable to political siren-songs about support of medical research. Learning something about how we went about trying to understand obesity may make it easier to assess the press releases about the "wars" that are being declared against various diseases, and the probable effect of massive infusions of money on when the enemy is likely to surrender.

one
Night Eating

I am fifty-three years old, a psychiatrist, and a teacher in a medical school. I am not now, and never have been, obese—nor are any of my close friends or relatives. In fact, until shortly before my chance involvement with obesity, I had no real interest in the subject. Yet for twenty-two years now obesity has been my major medical interest, the object of the largest part of my research effort, and the source of my greatest therapeutic satisfactions and bitterest therapeutic failures.

The path to my involvement with obesity was a circuitous one, through college and medical school, military service and psychiatric training, and I shall not recount it here. Ultimately I ended up at the New York Hospital with the opportunity to do clinical investigation. There were so few such opportunities for a psychiatrist in those days that I was happy to work on whatever research problem was presented to me. And since ours was a psychosomatic research group, and since migraine and ulcer and the rest of the psychosomatic disorders had already been assigned to others, obesity fell to my lot by a process of elimination. But within a few days I was fully engrossed in the subject.

Since obesity is so common, and since it had not previously been studied at the New York Hospital, I soon found myself in great demand, and soon was treating a fairly large number of obese people. Obesity, which means excessive fatness, is usually associated with people who are some twenty percent heavier than their "desirable" weights as calculated by the standard height/weight tables. But the body weight of most of the people with whom I worked far exceeded this figure of twenty percent; they were the massively obese.

One of the first features of obese people which caught my attention was the bland appearance which often overlay their intense suffering. Since the stereotype of the jolly fat man was still, even then, widely accepted, I began to think of starting my research with a consideration of this suffering and its relationship to its apparent denial by the sufferers. Both were well exemplified in my very first obese patient, Maxine Wilkins.

In the first place, Maxine had never even thought of treatment for her obesity. Yet at age 16 she weighed 220 pounds and was gaining at a rate of nearly ten pounds a month. With her small frame and five-foot figure, this weight made her appear, if not quite grotesque, at least matronly. Her severe black dress and chubby expressionless face, with black hair tightly drawn into a bun at the back of her head, gave her the appearance of a little old woman, from whom all the life had been drained.

Initially she said nothing about her obesity. She had been brought to the hospital by her mother because she had had attacks of excruciating pain in her abdomen. These pains, which had been increasing, had almost ended her schooling and now required morphine. The referring doctor's note, which also did not mention obesity, told the story that had become Maxine's standard reply to questions about her life: "Maxine is always happy, sociable, good in school work, has plenty of dates. Her family relationships are excellent."

In the course of learning about her abdominal pains, I asked Maxine what sort of things made her nervous and how she thought these might be related to her pain. With a sweet smile she told me that the other doctor who had seen her in the hospital had said she was to come to the psychiatric clinic because she was nervous. She said that while it was true that she had been nervous about seeing him, she hardly ever felt nervous at other times and didn't believe the nervousness could have anything to do with her pains. But she quickly added that she was quite willing to accept my advice if I felt there was a connection.

"Do you really think that nervousness could be causing the pain?" she asked. "I mean, it seems to me quite silly, though I suppose you know from studying the various cases, just how nervousness and worry could cause pain. . . ."

With a pretty smile she said that things were going very well in her life. She enjoyed her school work and regretted that her illness was keeping her from attending school and participating in its many fascinating activities. The illness had not, however, interfered with her social life to any great extent. She still went out on frequent dates, visited with her girl friends, and spent very happy hours at home. Home was, in fact, the center of her life, and the evenings with her family were pure delight. She and her sister played cards with their parents; she would listen to the ball game on the radio with her father; and her mother would play the piano and sing. The father had recently bought a recording machine, ". . . and we use it quite a lot for enjoyment." Enjoyment, it developed, was singing: "Just the three of us, Mother, Matilda, and me. And sometimes Daddy chimes in. He sings off key, but he enjoys it. Usually he takes care of the recording machine and lets us sing to our hearts' content." Throwing herself into the account with a radiant smile, Maxine assured me, "I think I have just about the best family in the whole world."

Since she did not admit to any problems, I was somewhat
surprised when Maxine readily agreed to psychiatric treatment. I would have been less surprised after my first few
months at our clinic, when I had heard similar presentations by
other obese people.

I remember facing the beginning of that treatment with
some concern. But assured by my reading that such a patient
must certainly have emotional problems, I was prepared to
believe that this was the case. But how, I wondered, would
I get her to acknowledge these problems, let alone work on
them?

I need not have been concerned. Maxine arrived at our
first treatment interview wearing her sweet, reassuring smile.
Then she said, "I must start off by confessing that I didn't
tell the truth about all the questions you asked me. One of
the things you asked me about was girl friends and things
like that, and I said that I had them. But I don't. And I
never had a date with a boy."

There had been a time, years before, when she had felt
that things had been as happy as she had described them
to me. She remembered as a little girl singing with her mother
and sister, playing cards with her parents, and days when
". . . Mother was carefree and not nervous . . . ," and
". . . Daddy used to take us out to dinner every week. . . .
But things changed after he got the job as a salesman.
That was four years ago. He used to take money from his
company fund, you know, to pay for food and medicines.
It was only for necessities. I mean my father *is* a grand man.
And then he would have to return the money at the end
of the week. That was always a terrible time. The whole family
would be up late on Thursday night trying to decide how
much of the money he should bring back."

Once the decision had been made, mother and daughters
would scatter on Friday morning, each visiting those neighbors
from whom she felt she had the best chance of borrowing.
They would return before the father went to work and give
him the money, which he would then use to replace what
he had appropriated. On Friday evening they would deliberate

how to make token repayments to the neighbors in an effort to keep these sources of support open.

"This went on all summer and then into the fall. All of us believed that by Christmas time things would get straightened out, and I kept looking forward to Christmas and praying for it to come. But then Christmas came, and things were just the same. It was dreadful. We just didn't know which way to turn."

Gradually this state of indebtedness became a way of life for the family and the central theme of its long, anxiety-ridden discussions. The small income the father earned from commissions was not enough to support the family's way of life, and the chronic borrowing gradually isolated them from the community. Maxine and her sister became increasingly uneasy in their contacts with neighbors, even contacts not related to borrowing money. Finally, her older sister took what appeared to be the only course that might bring some permanent relief. At the age of 17 she left school to take a job.

Maxine's main reaction to this event was shame, and she found it harder than ever to face the neighbors. "And I also felt just terrible that I wasn't helping the family the way Matilda was. So I used to try to help her by washing and ironing her clothes and doing little things for her."

At first Matilda enjoyed the relief her salary afforded the family, and basked in the increased attention she received and in the favors Maxine did for her. Then the family gradually adjusted to the new and higher income, and the cycle was repeated. The father's income began to fall off. Matilda began to get bitter. "She says it wouldn't be so bad if things were getting better. But they aren't. As long as the money comes in, Daddy won't change. She thought of stopping work so that he would have to earn some money, but. . . ."

As Maxine became progressively isolated from people outside the family, she turned more and more to Matilda, and for a time the two were close. Then Matilda realized that by taking a job she had not really changed the situation, and it began to be clear to her how she was being taken advantage of. She became demanding. The sisters began to argue over the increasing demands Matilda made of Maxine. Maxine began to feel exploited herself and refused her services; Matilda would remind her that she had been forced to leave school to work and support the family, and the least that Maxine could do was to help her in the few small things she asked.

The sisters continued to sleep in the same bed as they had since childhood, and here they would sometimes discuss the turmoil in which they were living. One evening they were discussing their father, soon after he had taken a job as a traveling salesman, which kept him away from home most of the time. "Last night Matilda had a premonition that Daddy had died, and she told me about it while we were lying in bed. Mother heard her talking and came in and made her tell about her premonition. It upset Mother just terribly, and she began to cry and scream, and then we all ended up crying. It seems like everybody in our family is always worried about everybody else."

Long before the pains had begun, Maxine had been considering some way out. "I don't deserve to be cared for the way my parents care for me, when they are so much in debt and so upset about it. It's impossible to do well in school feeling the way I do, and the girls seem so young and silly. I might as well leave—or commit suicide. I think of suicide a lot, particularly when I'm in bed at night, but I've never had the courage to go through with it."

What was the relationship of this turmoil to her weight? Maxine wasn't sure. She thought that her weight had been about normal before the troubles began, when she was about 12 years old. She did remember having been a "chubby" child. But the years that had been so filled with distress were blank as far as her weight was concerned. "I was really surprised when the doctor weighed me and I found out that I weighed 220 pounds. I didn't know how that had happened. I knew I was eating more than usual, but I would just say 'What's the use?' and go on. There's so much I'm not aware of, I don't know whether I realized that I was becoming heavy or not." It was not even clear she knew her over-eating was causing her overweight.

As I reviewed these notes, they clearly demonstrated the pain behind the bland appearance. It was the same pain I was seeing in so many obese people. A study focused on this discrepancy might have some merit in debunking the stereotype of the jolly fat man; but by this time it seemed increasingly important to focus on more specific topics. I was beginning to see other obese patients whose relations with their parents had much in common with those of Maxine. So I examined the notes on these relationships to try to understand them as fully as possible.

One central theme was the emphasis on family "closeness." In Maxine's family both daughters had been discouraged from having outside social interests, even before the financial troubles had made this inevitable. Within this confined family system the influence of each of the parents was enhanced.

It became unmistakably clear that one of Maxine's major ways of coping was to identify with her mother. And her mother was a huge woman, 275 pounds, with the same bland manner as her daughter. She denied any difficulties at home, dismissed her own obesity with only a hint of martyred self-sufficiency, as "just glands," and corroborated Maxine's initial story that the girl had a happy and sociable life. She even accepted therapy when it was offered to her, and attended faithfully for two or three months. She began treatment by shedding her mask, much as Maxine had done. She acknowledged what she saw as insuperable family problems. And she wept. According to the psychiatrist who saw her, that was about all she did during her treatment: She would begin to cry as soon as she entered the office, and cried almost uninterruptedly until the time was up. Nothing that her psychiatrist did would interrupt the flow of tears. Eventually they agreed to terminate the treatment, despairing of ever being able to get beyond her tears.

Maxine's intense self-consciousness seemed a direct reflection of her mother's. "Mother has always said that a heavy person should keep in the background and not do anything that would call attention to herself. She doesn't dance at parties, or do anything like that; she feels she would be making a fool of herself. And I guess I feel the same way. I just feel ridiculous all the time."

Only when Maxine's treatment began to make her more independent of her family, and less likely to be caught up in the recurrent family turmoil, was her mother able to mobilize herself. Apparently desperate because of the threat to the integrity of the family, both mother and father began to lash out at the treatment. Their message was the same: Maxine's motives for coming to the hospital were not therapeutic but sexual.

"Mother has been teasing me again about coming in to the hospital. She said that I was just coming in because I liked you, and that it's disgusting. She said that she couldn't let me waste the family's money on carfare for this sort of silliness. She said, 'If you and Dr. Stunkard are so close, let him come out here to see you.'"

As Maxine persisted in treatment, and her independence grew, her mother's attacks mounted. "Now she says that the reason I'm coming in is either because I'm a hopeless case or because I'm after your body, and she wants to know which one it is. She just keeps telling me how disgusting it is. I am afraid that she won't let me keep coming in and I don't know what to do about it."

Mrs. Wilkins was so ineffectual that even her desperation about the loss of Maxine could not rouse her to terminate treatment. Not so with Mr. Wilkins. Maxine's father was a man with an extraordinary ability to get what he wanted, and he managed to live the life of a pampered princeling even in these improbable circumstances. A large handsome man, his overweight skillfully disguised by excellent tailoring, he extracted from his environment a remarkable series of indulgences. Only late in the treatment did an embarrassed Maxine reveal that "Daddy has breakfast in bed every morning when he's home." She accepted this as a perfectly reasonable way of life, and was upset only because ". . . he never shows any appreciation to Mother for going to this trouble. He just seems to take it for granted. It's nice to have a happy-go-lucky attitude and to enjoy things, but sometimes I *do* wish that Daddy would be more serious. Sometimes it even irritates me the way he goes on. Oh, I know I shouldn't say things like that."

Usually Maxine met her father's demands, just as her mother and sister did. Why did these three women continue to support and pamper this man? One possibility was that the drabness of the family's life was somehow made to seem worthwhile when they provided enjoyment for Daddy, because Daddy seemed to be the only member of the family who could really enjoy himself. And Maxine was more than a little attracted to this winsome rogue. In this inhibited, confused, and demoralized family, the father's lack of inhibitions, his ability to seek gratification for himself regardless of the consequences to others, exercised a kind of magic. Whatever he said or did, he seemed more than life-size.

What he said to Maxine often confirmed her mother's querulous judgments: "He was just terrible last night. My own father said that if he were a boy he wouldn't give me a second look. He said I was getting fatter by the minute, and the treatment wasn't helping me at all. He said that I would be a good candidate for a circus pretty soon."

Mr. Wilkins had other motives for not wanting family matters discussed outside the house. It was difficult to reconstruct just what had happened from the anguished reports of a frightened teenager, and much of what Maxine reported may have been fantasy. What she told me of were some unusual steps her father was taking in relation to her sexual inhibitions. On four or five occasions during one confusing month he brought home a young friend from work, plied Maxine with drink, told dirty jokes and indicated that he would look favorably upon her accommodating his friend. She froze and resisted.

I learned about most of these events only much later, for in contrast to his wife's ineffectual remonstrances, Mr. Wilkins had moved decisively to terminate Maxine's treatment. She came in one evening profoundly discouraged. "Daddy has been just terrible. He says that this isn't psychiatric treatment, it's lovemaking. And the doctor ought to come to my house, so he would have to pay the carfare. Mother just keeps sitting there saying that it's all so disgusting."

Two days later the letter came from Maxine, breaking off treatment: "Regardless of anything I may have said about my parents, I love them deeply and cannot continue to bring them pain. I feel that my parents have always tried to act in my best interests, regardless of how it might seem to me at the time. I deeply regret that this decision has become necessary. It may be due to my weakness, and if this is so, I deeply regret it."

That was to be the last I heard of Maxine, but her story reflected a pattern with which I was already growing familiar. Within the first few months at the New York Hospital I had seen several family constellations similar to that of the Wilkins family. Time and again I had been struck by how many young obese women reflected the dominant themes in Maxine's life.

To a remarkable degree obesity runs in families: 90 percent of the children of two obese parents are themselves obese, compared to only 10 percent of the children of non-obese parents. On the fertile soil of obesity there grew, with surprising regularity, the same discouraged identification with a demoralized, obese mother—and the same hopelessness. Often, far more often than I would have expected, I discovered also the intense, fantasy-ridden longing for salvation through the love of a handsome hero.

I was contemplating a research project in the general area of obesity, and as fascinating as these parallels were, they did not seem suitable topics for a study. I continued searching, and at one point thought of considering obesity as a family problem. But neither this nor other ideas satisfied me. Then, in the midst of my quandary, the answer came.

For some time a group of us had gathered each week to listen to recordings of our interviews with patients. I had recorded one interview with Maxine, during the troubled time shortly before she had broken off treatment. Concerned by what had happened, I asked my colleagues to discuss the problem.

The meeting began with a description of Maxine's background and the problem in treatment. Then we began to listen to the recording. Suddenly one of our group became upset, a young woman psychiatrist who was obese. Gasping for air, she rose from the circle and began to stagger out of the room. Puzzled, I followed her. She had reached the door and was opening it by the time I could talk with her. Her face mirrored anguish bordering on panic. Only reluctantly was she persuaded to come back to the room.

Finally, with the recorder turned off, she tried to explain to a baffled, solicitous group what had happened, what had precipitated her attack of acute anxiety. "It wasn't anything about the father. That was nothing. It was how that girl talked about the way she eats: Nothing for breakfast. She is never hungry at all in the morning. Then what it's like at night, how she can't seem to stop eating. Supper doesn't satisfy her, and she just goes on and on. She even gets up out of bed to eat . . . That's how I eat, and I never heard about it from anybody else in my whole life!"

For some time we discussed with the obese psychiatrist her reaction to the recording, and then moved on to the problem of the interrupted treatment. But the incident of the anxiety attack stuck in my mind. I could never forget that shock of recognition—the sudden realization that an eating pattern could be so much more meaningful to another obese woman than the lurid events we had been discussing. Here it seemed might be a topic suitable for careful investigation.

Did other obese patients show this pattern? I was quite sure that they did. But the careful dietary histories I had taken from each of my patients had focused on the amount and the kinds of foods eaten, and they had not paid any special attention to the pattern of eating. Nevertheless I seemed to remember patients telling me of skipping breakfasts and of eating at night. It was easy enough to find out. As each of my patients returned to the clinic, I asked them about their eating patterns. As so rarely happens, the questions were on target.

With a rush of recognition, the first patient I asked told me that she never ate breakfast, never snacked in the morning, and had little or no appetite for lunch. Then as the day wore on, particularly after supper, she ate more and more heavily. Occasionally she would even get up out of bed, go to the refrigerator and fix herself a sandwich. On such evenings her agitation and turmoil were unbearable.

The next obese patient also reported a lack of appetite for breakfast, eating heavily in the evening, and being upset at that time. With mounting enthusiasm, I posed the questions to each of the obese patients I was treating. I learned that if they ate in this pattern, they were well aware of it and only too ready to describe it. If they didn't eat in this manner, they were also quite well aware of the fact. There was nothing ambiguous; either the phenomenon was there or it was not.

The next steps were quite simple. If the phenomenon could be easily identified, how common was it? I made a list of my patients, and after questioning them wrote down which aspects of the phenomenon (which became known as "the night-eating pattern") were present. It was soon apparent that most of them exhibited three common characteristics: lack of appetite in the morning, over-eating in the evening, and combined agitation and insomnia. These held true for none of the non-obese patients.

As I explored the night-eating pattern further, however, a complication developed. Some patients said that although they were eating this way at present, they had not always done so. Others reported that they had eaten this way in the past, but were not doing so now. What made the difference? About this time one of my patients had an experience that helped to answer the question.

Maureen Reilly was a 29-year-old housewife. She had been referred to our clinic for treatment of obesity, which was causing frequent and severe attacks of inflammation in the veins of her legs. The eighth of ten living children, she remembered her mother with great bitterness for having, she was convinced, exploited her. Whatever the truth of these complaints, her childhood had been a time of hardship and deprivation. The father's sporadic employment never permitted the family more than a marginal existence.

At age 18 Mrs. Reilly had married the neighborhood alcoholic in an effort to escape her home environment. It was a jump from the frying pan into the fire, and she soon bitterly regretted it. But children followed, and she found herself enmeshed in inescapable obligations. Within eight years of her marriage she had added 100 pounds to her sturdy 5'6" frame, reaching a weight of 280. Her weight had stayed at this level for three years when she came to the clinic.

Mrs. Reilly's manner was pleasant and friendly, but her communication had an oddly impersonal quality. She was usually late for appointments, and her attendance was irregular.

When she came to the clinic she displayed a clear-cut night-eating pattern. She regularly awoke in the morning with no appetite and ate no breakfast and little lunch. Supper, in the early evening, was large, but only temporarily satisfying. During the rest of the evening, often until early morning, she nibbled at various foods distinguished mainly by their sweetness. She was unclear about why she ate at these times, but she thought it might be due to anxiety.

Her anxiety was most severe when she was alone, when she would worry about someone breaking into the house and harming her. The measures she took provided only partial relief: besides eating, she would have company in the house, and when alone, she would keep the radio and lights on. Sometimes the presence of her husband reassured her, but as often she would quarrel with him and then feel even more upset. She would stay up eating until midnight at least, and often until two or three in the morning. Throughout my early contact with her, she rarely slept more than four hours a night.

Just at the point when I was beginning my systematic inquiry into the night-eating pattern, Mrs. Reilly developed a recurrence of her phlebitis, which made it necessary for her to enter the hospital. Not surprisingly she greeted this development with relief and gladly laid down her domestic responsibilities.

Within a day her eating pattern changed strikingly. The

morning after she entered the hospital, she awoke with a desire
to eat breakfast, for the first time in months. She went on
to eat an average-sized lunch and a small supper, and had
no desire to eat during the evening or night. This absence
of night eating was all the more remarkable in that the pain
in her legs kept her awake much of the night during her first
week in the hospital. Thereafter she slept well, never complained of hunger, adhered with no difficulty to an 800-Calorie
diet, and lost 28 pounds in a month.

This marked change in her eating pattern was paralleled
by a great decrease in anxiety. In fact Mrs. Reilly seemed
more at ease than I had ever seen her. She attributed part
of the change in her eating pattern, and in her comfort, to
the presence of her roommate. "She keeps me feeling good
in the evenings by talking to me. Then I don't feel like eating."

Mrs. Reilly wanted very much to remain in the hospital,
and she used every conceivable stratagem to delay her discharge. Finally, reluctantly, she returned home. Within 24
hours the night-eating pattern had returned. The morning
after her arrival home she awoke with no appetite, did not
begin to eat until evening, and then stayed up until three
the next morning, nibbling. Her husband, who had stopped
drinking while she was in the hospital, began again as soon
as she returned home. The relations between them, which had
improved during her hospitalization, deteriorated rapidly.
During her first month home Mrs. Reilly regained ten pounds.

Was this then the reason for the apparent capriciousness
with which the night-eating pattern came and went? Was
it a response to life stress? And did it disappear, along with
the anxiety and agitation, when the stress was relieved? For
Mrs. Reilly the answer seemed to be "yes." When I asked
my other patients, they agreed.

Once I felt confident that there truly was a night-eating
pattern, the subsequent exploration followed almost automatically. It was largely a process of setting down the findings in a
way that made it easy to discover relationships between them. I
found none of any significance. The night-eating pattern
occurred in young and old, short and tall, slightly overweight

and severely obese. Over-all it occurred in 20 of the 25 obese patients, whom I was treating at that time.

However, one finding did stand out in bold relief: Five of the twenty-five patients did *not* show the night-eating pattern—and four of these five were losing weight. In fact they had lost a great deal of weight, from 45 to as much as 105 pounds. Of the twenty patients with the night-eating pattern, only two had lost as much.

Five patients with the night-eating pattern had lost lesser amounts of weight, from 20 to 30 pounds, and had then discontinued their diets. But these attempts at dieting were noteworthy. It looked as if the weight loss of four of them had occurred during a temporary remission in their night-eating pattern.

What about past efforts to lose weight? Four of the five patients without the night-eating pattern had been able to lose weight in the past. And only 11 of the 20 with the night-eating pattern had been successful.

One practical consequence was apparent. When the outcome of treatment is as uncertain as it is in obesity, it is useful to be able to predict which patients are likely to succeed. The night-eating pattern presaged failure, not success. But inasmuch as it indicated the outcome of treatment, it provided a useful diagnosis. It could spare obese people with a poor outlook for weight reduction another unhappy attempt at dieting, and another experience with failure. And limited treatment resources could be allocated to those most apt to benefit from them.

The difficulty in losing weight fascinated me. It was not something that began when these patients came to our clinic. Only 11 of the 20 night-eaters had successfully reduced at any time in their lives. These weight losses had been unusual events. How had the patients been able to accomplish them? What had happened when they did? I began to ask them more about these successful diets.

As I pursued this question, an engrossing story emerged. The night-eaters had been able to lose weight only at extraordinary cost. For eight of these eleven patients, weight loss had

been accompanied by disabling emotional illness! Recon-
structing the character of these illnesses long after the event
was difficult. They seemed to run the gamut of symptoms:
depression, fatigue, anxiety, feelings of futility. Furthermore,
the illnesses seemed to arise in a great variety of circumstances.
Clearly it was going to take time to understand these disorders.

At this point events brought home in a brutal manner the
emotional complications of dieting. One of my few patients
who seemed to be doing really well was a 49-year-old woman.
She had come with a variety of complaints: migraine headaches, generalized muscular aching, a nervous disorder of the
skin that she had had for 20 years, and depression. The fact
that she was obese and showed the night-eating pattern seemed
almost incidental.

The center of a large Italian family, Mrs. Rosselini had
years ago settled into a grim depressed mood, martyred and
long-suffering. Having decided to devote her life to her eight
children, she gained a measure of satisfaction by serving them
through the never-ending housework she knew so well. Before
she had passed the child-bearing age her older children were
already bringing their babies for her to look after. As the
years went by she became even busier, and even more
depressed.

I began seeing Mrs. Rosselini for weekly 45-minute psychotherapy sessions. At first all I heard were tired, repetitious
accounts of her symptoms and of her past experiences, most
of them unfavorable, with doctors. By the end of a month,
however, she began to speak of her home. Soon she was regal-
ing me with dramatic accounts of how she was mistreated
and how she suffered. Gradually she began to see that she
had collaborated in setting up her unenviable home life, and
began to explore the possibility of changing it.

For a beginning, Mrs. Rosselini began to refuse her
children when their demands struck her as excessive. And
she even asked them for help when her housework became
too demanding. She began to talk about the possibility of
getting out of the house, and her old dream of working in
a hospital as a nurse's aide was reborn. I was delighted by

these developments, and encouraged her to undertake activities that might foster her growing independence of her family. Then her family began to react against their mother's new-found freedom. I met with her eldest son and persuaded him to support her against this opposition.

Two months into her treatment, I spoke to Mrs. Rosselini about the possible benefits of weight reduction. I said I hoped she would try to lose some weight. She was enthusiastic about the idea and began to diet at once. In the next two months her weight fell from 183 to 170 pounds. And her other symptoms just seemed to melt away. Her depression lifted. Her muscles stopped aching. Her skin stopped itching. Her headaches went away.

Only gradually did it begin to dawn on me that Mrs. Rosselini was becoming unusually active. So few of my patients were doing well that I didn't want to question what seemed like a therapeutic triumph. But finally I could no longer ignore her accounts of exuberant and seemingly tireless activities, her decreasing need for sleep, her increasingly seductive dress. I began to be concerned that she was becoming manic. Then the bottom dropped out.

One day about four months after we had begun treatment, Mrs. Rosselini arrived at the clinic in a tight-fitting, low-cut, black dress. Her gray hair, newly blued, was piled in cascades upon her head; she was wearing a pearl necklace, a pearl bracelet, pearl earrings. Breathlessly she told me of further weight loss since her last visit and beamed at my approval. She asked if she had lost enough weight to satisfy me. Puzzled and uneasy, I asked her what she meant.

She began a tortured account of what lay behind the dramatic changes in her life. At our very first interview she had formed the notion that I must be in love with her, and everything that happened afterwards confirmed this belief. Why else, she argued, would I have disapproved of the mistreatment she suffered at the hands of her family? Why else would I have met with her eldest son to encourage the family to lighten her load? Why else would I have wanted her to be slimmer and more attractive? She had done what I had

asked; she had lost weight. Now it was up to me. She was
ready to go away with me. She was ready to marry me if
I wished. To my question about her family, she said that
she had no more worries about what her family would think.
She was free of her family. She had suffered for them; now
it was time for her to live for herself.

I fumbled out some poor response, mortified by my
blindness.

Mrs. Rosselini's disillusionment was prompt and profound. She could not believe that she had so misread my
intentions. She burst into tears. She asked me again to take
her away. Then she left the office.

Mrs. Rosselini did not keep her next appointment. She
did not return to the clinic until her family brought her, three
weeks later. By then she was severely depressed. She told me
that after her last visit she had been very frightened, and
had cried almost constantly. She said she was sleeping poorly
and had nightmares in which strange men attacked and
robbed her. Her speech and actions were slow; she professed
no interest in anything. She had given up any effort to take
care of her house.

Unlike most persons suffering from depression, Mrs. Rosselini did not express any ideas of guilt or self-condemnation.
If anyone were to blame, it was I. Her reaction, she maintained, was a perfectly normal one. How else was a woman
to act when she was abandoned by the man she loved? But
even now, she said, there was still time for me to rescue her.

Mrs. Rosselini continued to come to the clinic for a few
more months, unhappy, depressed, accusing, asking if I had
changed my mind. Then her family took her to another doctor.
From then on I learned about her only through the courtesy
of several of the doctors whom she consulted. Apparently she
remained depressed for more than a year, during which time
she went through an extraordinary assortment of medical
treatments, none of which provided much relief. Some were
psychiatric—psychotherapy, electroshock, three months in a
psychiatric hospital. Others were surgical. During one six-
month period she underwent three major operations, under-

taken in large part at her insistence, for conditions such as hernia, that were not causing her any discomfort. In addition she was treated by internists and general practitioners.

Eventually Mrs. Rosselini's sufferings restored the sympathy and concern of her family. Its members began to treat her once again with the consideration they had abandoned when she had tried to assert her independence. By the time her more severe depressive symptoms had abated, she had already returned to her drab, colorless existence. She remained mildly depressed; her muscles began to ache again, her skin resumed its itching, her migraine returned. Her weight rose once again to over 180 pounds.

Mrs. Rosselini's breakdown had a powerful effect on how I viewed the complications of weight reduction. No longer were they episodes in a remote past, academic matters whose details had already slipped from the memory of my informants. These complications were now a burning problem.

two
Dieting and Depression

It had taken quite a while to decide upon the topic for my first research effort—night-eating. Not so the second. It arose from a concrete and pressing problem: to learn about the kind of emotional disturbance which had afflicted Mrs. Rosselini when she had tried to lose weight. For I was beginning to hear about similar troubles from other obese people. If this were a danger, it was one we had to know about. I was concerned not only for myself, but for all of the other physicians treating obese people, lest we actually add to the heavy burdens they were already carrying.

This next study started with an article of faith: that there was a consistent pattern to the emotional upsets I had observed in some of my patients when they attempted to diet. Perhaps

25

a treatment program would evolve from learning more about this pattern.

I began by utilizing the natural history approach, that is, spending a great deal of time with each of the 25 obese patients I was then treating, and trying to find out everything I could about their past experiences with dieting. I tried to learn how often each one had dieted, how long the diets had lasted, why they had been undertaken, how the patient felt during the diet, and why he or she had stopped—in short anything that might throw light on the kind of difficulty Mrs. Rosselini had encountered.

My questions about the night-eating pattern had already revealed that eight of the twenty-five patients had experienced an emotional upset when they dieted. But these emotional upsets didn't fit any of the standard diagnoses. Depression was present, but so were anxiety and fatigue and feelings of futility. It took time before one fact became conspicuous: the diet which had ushered in the emotional disturbance had not been undertaken casually. In each case, it had had profound implications for the patient; the expectations had far exceeded what might reasonably have been hoped for from a diet. In more than one instance these expectations had been inadvertently fostered by a physician, sometimes by me, sometimes by another. There was at least some small comfort in learning that Mrs. Rosselini's illness was not unprecedented, and that other physicians had similarly blundered.

One patient's illness was particularly interesting, since I knew her physician and was able to compare his recollection of events with hers. (He had had no idea that his patient had become ill while dieting, and was stunned to learn of the part he had played.)

Maria Malone was a 34-year-old housewife who weighed 214 pounds when she came to our clinic, complaining of obesity and migraine headaches. Her obesity had been slowly increasing since her adolescence, except for two attempts at weight reduction. The first attempt had been uneventful, the second disastrous, ushering in a severe emotional disturbance.

Mrs. Malone was the eldest of two daughters, raised in

an authoritarian Irish-immigrant family. Much of her childhood had been spent in useless competition with her younger
sister, who had become their parents' favorite because of her
sickly childhood, her conforming behavior, and her supposedly
greater abilities. After graduating from high school, Mrs.
Malone had made an unsuccessful attempt to study art and
then had become a secretary in a large industrial organization.
There she had formed a strong attachment to a fellow worker.
He must have been a curious man—bitter, rebellious, remarkably passive, 12 years her senior. She had idolized him
throughout five years of a platonic friendship. And when he
finally proposed marriage, she accepted at once, thrilled by
this proposal and grateful to him for his motives for marrying
her. He was willing to marry her, he announced, out of pure
altruism. His goal was to develop her potential and to make
her over into the wonderful person he was sure she could
become.

As could have been forecast, their illusions did not sur-
vive the first months of marriage. They soon bogged down in
a life of intense mutual dependency, bitter with recrimina-
tions about the supposedly inadequate care each was giving
the other. Mrs. Malone gave birth to three children and raised
them while going about her housewifely duties "as blank as
that wall." Periodically she would break away into exuberant
participation in community activities.

She had been worried for some years by the apparent
attraction between her sister and her husband. One day she
returned home to find them locked in a passionate embrace.
Her immediate reaction was, "the world is falling apart," and
she became panicky and disorganized. Her husband and sister,
upset and chastened, made every effort to reassure Mrs. Malone about their love for her and the casualness of their relationship. But she was inconsolable. A week or two later, having
assured herself that her husband and children were in the
next room, she turned on the gas in the kitchen.

At this point her husband became alarmed and took
her to the leading physician in the area, reputedly a wise
and compassionate man. From what I knew about him this

reputation was fully justified. Mrs. Malone was impressed, as others had been before her, by his kindness and understanding. She left his office after her first visit feeling much better. During her second visit, when he had learned more about the situation, he recommended that she return for weekly talks to help her understand some of her difficulties. When she protested that the family could not afford the expense, he replied that he would be willing to see her without charge. Puzzled, she asked him how this was possible. His reply, which loomed larger in later events, burned into her memory: "I'll be getting as much out of this as you."

At the time this doctor was becoming interested in psychotherapy and was selecting a few of his more articulate and troubled patients for regular interviews. Later, when I asked him about these events, he vaguely remembered having offered Mrs. Malone free weekly visits, but he had been quite unaware of the significance this offer had held for her. She came to his office once a week for about two months, and then stopped. She said she found she was, for no apparent reason, unable to talk to him. By this time she was over the acute anxiety and, so she thought, "back to my old self."

Several weeks after Mrs. Malone stopped seeing the doctor, she again had a sudden upset. It occurred when a neighbor brought up the subject of adultery. Mrs. Malone found herself becoming confused and excited. Unsure of what was happening to her, she hurriedly left her neighbor to try to straighten out her thoughts. These thoughts began to converge on one topic: a love affair with the doctor. As she went back over her talks with him, his remark, "I'll be getting as much out of this as you," began to assume a special meaning. Perhaps, she imagined, he had just been too shy to come right out and tell her his intentions. If that were the case, she decided to give him the opportunity. She called for another appointment.

But as soon as Mrs. Malone entered the doctor's office, her courage failed her. She became embarrassed and was unable to tell him why she had come. In fact, she had trouble saying anything. For a time the physician tried fruitlessly to help her to talk. Then, drumming his fingers on the table, he noted that she had not had a physical examination for some time. He suggested that it might be well to see how she was doing, and then proceeded to examine her. For Mrs. Malone the examination was a confirmation of all her hopes. Here was a man too shy to express his desires in a forthright way. But through his actions he left no doubt about his intentions. She returned home in high spirits.

When I spoke with the physician about these events, he vaguely remembered what had happened. He had been impressed first with Mrs. Malone's highly articulate account of her problems, and later with her growing difficulty in talking. He remembered feeling some relief when she had stopped coming for treatment, since things had been going so slowly. He did recall carrying out the physical examination, but none of the circumstances surrounding it, and learned of her reaction with the greatest chagrin.

For the next six months Mrs. Malone walked on air. Despite the fact that she did not see the physician during this time, she felt that "emotionally he was always with me, no matter where I was or what I did . . . It made me feel full, a terrible, pleasant sense of fullness." Much of her time was spent in romantic fantasies of how the doctor would come to rescue her from her drab and meaningless existence. In her mind, the physical examination had been not only an inarticulate expression of his sexual desire, but evidence as well of his wish that she become more attractive by losing weight. Exuberantly, and without the slightest difficulty, Mrs. Malone embarked on a reducing diet that brought her weight down from 225 to 175 pounds in less than six months.

During this period she seemed to have limitless energy, sailing through her formerly burdensome household activities with feelings of delight and accomplishment. She increased her participation in community activities and even resumed her old adolescent interest in painting. "It was different from the way things had been before. I had real feelings—love, and hate, and envy, and lust and passion." And for several weeks she luxuriated in her fantasies, with no concrete idea of when

her rescue was to take place. She formed a vague notion that
it would occur when her dieting had made her into the beautiful woman the physician's physical examination had revealed
as the object of his desire. This notion became more concrete
as her weight continued to melt away.

Then Mrs. Malone became troubled. With increasing
apprehension she watched her weight decline towards the limit
that would signal the transformation of her fantasy into reality.
By the time it had reached 175 pounds, she could no longer
keep her ideas to herself. With many misgivings, she gave
her husband a much modified account of what she thought
had been happening between her and the doctor.

Mr. Malone was furious. Exploding into a barrage of
oaths, he dragged his wife out to their car and drove recklessly
to the physician's office. Striding past the patients in the
waiting area, he burst into the examining room with Mrs.
Malone in his wake, shook his finger at the physician and
told him in a loud dramatic voice never to see his wife again.
Then, sulking and silent, he took her out of the office and
drove home.

Dazed but relieved, Mrs. Malone spent the next day
ruminating over the events of the confrontation—her husband's
anger, the doctor's bewilderment, and her own sense of having
been nothing more than a bystander. She finally satisfied
herself that she had given her husband ample warning. She
could now proceed without guilt or fear of recrimination. She
telephoned the doctor and began by saying that she had been
thinking about her husband's reaction. Then she added that
perhaps he was right and that it might be better if they did
not meet again. To her surprise the doctor agreed.

"I felt devastated, as if the most wonderful person in the
world had died. It was a terrible sense of loss." For weeks
she suffered from what she described as "emptiness," and her
ebullient overactivity gave way to indolence and apathy. She
lost interest in her personal appearance, kept wearing the same
old black dress long after it had become dirty and wrinkled.
She even stopped wearing make-up, and neglected her hair.
Household chores again overwhelmed her. She could feed the

children and get them off to school; and that was all.

As Mrs. Malone recovered from the initial shock of disillusionment, she began to be oppressed by "guilt," by "a horror of what I had been ready to do." This horror was intensified as she came to realize that the whole affair might have existed solely in her imagination. For months she languished in a state of morbid introspection, contemplating her depravity, "feeling I was wrong again, like I always used to be." It was the end of a year before most of these symptoms had subsided, and once again Mrs. Malone was back to her old, drab life. Her weight gradually increased to 225 pounds.

As I reviewed the emotional illnesses of my obese patients, it became clear not only that they were closely connected with a diet, but also that the diet had a special significance, closely related to attempts to achieve independence. Here was the same kind of conflict, between the desire for independence and the fear of it, which had loomed so large in the life of Maxine Wilkins. The diet, it appeared, gained its heightened significance as a symbol of independence; to diet and become thin was to become free. And the diets that portended trouble seemed to be those that coincided with a decision to break off an important dependency relationship.

If these assessments were even partially correct, they suggested certain precautions it would be well to take in treating Mrs. Malone. Her past history showed that she was vulnerable to dieting and to misinterpreting her relationship with a physician. She was also very dependent upon her husband, despite her denials and despite the bitterness of her complaints about him. I decided to support her efforts toward independence, but very cautiously.

Early in treatment both Mrs. Malone and I became aware of the dangers that faced us. She came to our clinic at about the time that I was starting my systematic inquiry into the complications of dieting. We spent a good deal of time during her early visits in the clinic discussing these complications. We emerged from this inquiry with respect for the troubles that we could get into. But there were also some positive accomplishments. Talking about her illness seemed to help Mrs. Malone. Until then she had been unable to think about it with any objectivity and instead had viewed it as an ominous period of confusion and chaos. She seemed to gain strength from discussing the illness, getting clear on just what had happened, on the chronology of events, on the limits of her guilt. One of the major benefits of psychotherapy for someone who has undergone a mental illness may be this simple one, of helping to bring order out of chaos, of getting clear with another person on just what did happen.

The next step was to help Mrs. Malone express her anger towards her husband and to help her understand why she felt so angry. Then, very cautiously, we attempted to help her take some small, realistic steps toward greater independence. By consolidating her many community activities, for instance, she was able to take on greater responsibility in those she chose to continue.

One of my major goals in treating Mrs. Malone was to stay out of trouble. This was certainly a come-down from the grand goals of a few years before. In psychoanalytic training our greatest scorn had been reserved for what we called "melioristic" approaches to treatment. Nothing less than thorough-going personality reorganization would satisfy us as a worthy goal. And now here I was adopting a melioristic approach if ever there was one. And it seemed quite appropriate.

Over a period of a year and a half we succeeded in staying out of trouble. She lost some weight, from the 214 pounds which she brought to our clinic to 190 pounds. Her migraine headaches stopped almost completely. And when we finally terminated treatment, it was for a reason I had never expected. *Mr.* Malone became ill. As his wife showed a slow but steady increase in her ability to manage her affairs, and she became less dependent upon him, Mr. Malone became frightened, then angry. He finally developed a peptic ulcer. In time the ulcer became unmanageable; and he was forced to spend longer and longer periods in the hospital.

The origins of this difficulty seemed clear, and Mrs. Malone and I spoke about it at length, trying to see how her increasing independence might be made less threatening to him. But he was not in a position to accept help from his wife. And he adamantly refused both her and my suggestions that he seek psychotherapy. So Mrs. Malone eventually gave up treatment and went back to a somewhat less driven dependency upon her husband. Mr. Malone recovered from his ulcer. And they went on—unhappy, still mutually recriminatory, but perhaps a bit more comfortable than before.

This was my most impressive experience with the interlocking neuroses of marital partners. It was not to be the last. I feel sure, from the vantage point of today's knowledge about family therapy, that a great deal more could have been done for the Malones had I felt free to treat Mr. Malone along with his wife. I believe he might have welcomed this kind of help, which he could have seen as a way of rehabilitating his sick wife. And small shifts in the equilibrium of the two might well have accomplished as much for their adjustment as a major personality reorganization of Mrs. Malone would have. For then she would not have been forced to choose between living with a disconsolate husband or abandoning him.

But the teaching of the day frowned upon a psychiatrist treating both husband and wife. And it disparaged the results of such treatment as "superficial . . . environmental manipulation, . . . mere social work." So I did what I had been taught to do, and learned more about the inadequacy of our methods. This learning was to serve me in good stead in my treatment of Phyllis Baker.

Of all the patients who taught me about dieting and depression, Phyllis Baker stands out as my best teacher. Like Maria Malone, she had undergone a severe emotional illness during an earlier attempt at dieting. As with Maria Malone, I started treatment well aware of the possible dangers and took particular care to avoid them. What happened thus seems particularly significant.

Phyllis Baker was one of the most obese patients I had yet treated. Only five feet tall, she weighed 240 pounds when she arrived at our clinic to say that her eating was out of control and her weight increasing rapidly. Her appearance was remarkable. She was a woman of 22 years, who appeared to be in her middle teens. Her enormous body was covered by a dirty, cheap, cotton print dress that was stained and wrinkled. Perched atop this mammoth body, her small and striking head was dominated by a large aquiline nose and a mass of unkempt, red-blonde hair which swept out from her head in an untidy mass. On what must have been the apex of her massive breasts, two buttons advertised the Liberal Party candidate for mayor in the forthcoming election.

Phyllis was obviously very anxious as I invited her to sit down. Her hands were in almost constant motion, and she kept wringing them in the motion of distress of women three times her age. When she spoke her voice quavered and broke. She was barely able to tell me why she had come to the clinic.

Obesity was only one of her problems. Equally serious, she felt, was her problem with alcohol. She spent almost every evening in bars, drank to drunkenness every other night, and found herself in all manner of distasteful and dangerous circumstances as a result. She also said she was very nervous in crowds or groups of people. Her appearance made all this quite believable.

As Phyllis unfolded her many problems, I began to share her sense of being overwhelmed. Yet she had been working, supporting herself, getting by. She must have had some hope that she could be helped. "What," I asked, "do you hope to get out of treatment?"

She didn't hesitate. "To become a worthwhile member of the human race." I said that I gathered she did not feel that way now. She replied, "I feel the farthest thing from it."

The desolation and horror chilled me. "How *do* you feel about yourself?"

Again she did not hesitate. "I think of myself as a great mass of gray-green, amorphous material. Then at times I feel like a sloth. And just now, when I got up on the examining table, I felt like an elephant."

I had rarely heard anyone, even patients hospitalized

for mental illness, condemn themselves with the intensity of Phyllis Baker. She felt that people were watching her. Perhaps they really were; perhaps she just imagined it. But the self-loathing accorded fully with her complaint that things seemed unreal much of the time. Her account was as unsettling as her appearance.

Phyllis Baker's memories of childhood were marked by almost unrelieved gloom. She was one of several illegitimate children, who, with an older brother, had been left in the care of a widow, whom she had come to know as "Mother." She had few memories before those of her first day at school. Soon after she arrived, still excited by the occasion, she was picked out of her class by the school nurse, who found lice in her hair and dutifully announced the fact to the class. She was sent home with a note to her mother to wash her hair in kerosene.

Many children have been concerned by what the neighbors think of their family. For Phyllis, the problem was what the vice squad thought. When she was seven years old, the vice squad took a special interest in the "rooming house" which was her mother's ostensible source of income. Their concern was for the moral influence on the children. The problem was "solved" by getting her mother to marry one of the "boarders," a quiet and ineffectual man. Phyllis said, "When I found out about this, I was overwhelmed by his generosity and goodness. He just did it for me. He didn't have any other reason. The marriage was never consummated." It was only later, while she was in treatment, that Phyllis discovered that this was not the case, and her disillusionment increased.

Phyllis' own sexual experiences began at age five, when she thought she had had sexual intercourse with a boy. She *knew* that she had had intercourse by age six, for her sex play was with teenage boys, ". . . and it hurt terribly when they got into me." By then she had been discovered by her brother, who kept threatening to tell her mother. She had spent sleepless nights wondering what was going to happen to her, and remembered lying in bed waiting for her heart to stop beating.

Twelve was a critical age for Phyllis, the year when her periods started, and fear of pregnancy stopped her sexual activity. She had looked forward to this time, hoping that abstinence might make her more comfortable. The opposite had occurred. The severe, sometimes crippling anxiety that had struck me so forcibly during our first meeting had begun then. It was present only some of the time, but the fact that it began at a time that she had hoped would bring an end to her fearfulness had been profoundly disillusioning. She had begun to over-eat, and had become obese.

We spent a great deal of time trying to understand her over-eating and the period when it had begun. She felt that part of the explanation lay in the family's attitude toward food. "They always impressed on me as a child that if you eat, you are secure. That's one sign of security. I remembered so often my father saying, 'Well, we'll never starve. We've always got food on the table.' I suppose that's why I get so much pleasure out of food, and why I feel so strong when I'm eating."

At times Phyllis insisted that she did not over-eat because of hunger. She had feelings that others might interpret as hunger—like emptiness in the upper part of her abdomen—but she didn't consider this hunger. "It's emptiness, just general emptiness, and it goes away completely when I eat." It was always hard for me to believe that her feelings of emptiness in the abdomen differed from what other people called hunger. But her eating experiences certainly differed. "It's like I'm in love with food when I'm eating." Afterwards she felt remorse. "When I finish, I really hate food, After I've eaten, lots of times I feel sick. But when I'm eating, I feel good."

When Phyllis had begun to over-eat, at age 12, it was mostly during the day. But by the time she began treatment she was in the night-eating pattern, which was unusual in view of the large amounts of alcohol she consumed and the various foods available in bars.

The age of 12 had been memorable also for "the big family split." For some time a boarder, not her father, had tried to take on the disciplining of Phyllis' increasingly delinquent brother. Eventually the boarder's beatings led to violent arguments between Phyllis' mother and father, which culminated in a fight, during which her mother knocked her father down. Bitterly the family split into two factions, Phyllis, her mother, and the boarder in one, her father and brother in the other. They divided the house into halves, and for years thereafter the members of each faction religiously stayed in their assigned part of the house.

Despite the enormous difficulties under which she labored, Phyllis had done surprisingly well in her school work. As graduation from high school had approached, she had begun to look upon college as an escape from her trouble-ridden home. When her application to a nearby junior college was accepted, she was elated and joyfully prepared to leave home. Her mother's response was uncompromising opposition. Ordinary work was good enough for most people; why did Phyllis feel above it? She might as a starter, her mother suggested, begin to repay all the sacrifices she had made for a daughter who was not even hers. When gentler measures did not suffice, her mother began to berate Phyllis for her arrogance and cruelty in presuming to set herself above the family.

But Phyllis went nonetheless; and the first few weeks away from home were exciting ones. She embarked on a series of self-improvement measures, prominent among them her first serious attempt at dieting. In six months she lost 70 pounds.

What happened thereafter never became very clear. The work she undertook to support herself took time away from her school assignments. School was much harder than she had expected. Her classmates were no more friendly than they had been in high school. She failed her mid-year exams. Six months after leaving home Phyllis returned, frightened and defeated.

She said that she had suffered at that time from a "minor depression," and preferred not to talk about it. But what she did say revealed no "minor" depression. For a year and a half she had been unable to work. She stayed home, crying, depressed, unconcerned about her appearance—feeling futile, apathetic, and without hope. She regained the weight she had lost, and with a measure of relief, surrendered the conduct of her life to her mother.

The results were not quite what she expected. Accepting Phyllis as a colleague, her mother took her along on nightly rounds of pub-crawling. Life was soon dominated by heavy drinking and sex. Neither was satisfying. For Phyllis a drinking bout was precipitated by feelings quite different from the sense of "emptiness" that started her eating. "Rage," and to a lesser extent "frustration" were ". . . what started me drinking. When I get started with a bottle, I have a wonderful feeling of defiance. The hell with the whole world. I don't need anybody or anything, and nobody can do a damned thing to me. Screw 'em all."

Phyllis had been about 16 when she first became aware of a new kind of problem, new feelings that were later to cause her great distress. They began as romantic fantasies. "I would spend all of my time in my room, just lying there and thinking about being a man. I would be a sailor and travel all over the world. Or I would be a famous card player and go to Monte Carlo, and play cards, and rescue a damsel in distress. Particularly, most of all, I wanted to be a famous pitcher in the big leagues." Often the daydreams were quite focused. "I wanted a penis. I wanted to be a tall, dark, handsome man with a penis."

Phyllis had bridged the gap from fantasy to action in the sexual sphere, as in many others, with alcohol. All she had to do was to be present in a bar, in the security of the half-light, get drunk, and let things happen. She would be picked up by a woman and taken off, with no initiative on her part. Then, when the love-making started, "I come alive. I remember so well the first time. Afterwards I feel so proud . . . gay . . . light-hearted . . . responsible." There was no similarity to the fearful, furtive sex with men. Here was real excitement, ". . . the excitement of giving of myself, of making love, of giving love. I adore being allowed to play the male part."

We discussed at length what it meant to love women and how she had felt about it. "No, I don't feel like a man then, even though I do feel like I'm doing a man's work. I feel I have to satisfy the women." And she ruminated over male and female, man and woman. "It's not like being a man, and it's not like being a woman. I guess it sounds kind of wacky, but what it's really like is a boy doing a man's work."

Once, many months into treatment, Phyllis began to talk about her sexual feelings with increased intensity. It was quite important, somehow, to tell me about them. At first she could not, but finally she said, "I'm not sure about wanting to take care of other women. I think that's all too noble. I just want to get my head in between her legs. That's what gives me real peace! Being walled off, and walled in, and restful."

Gradually, as the months passed and Phyllis kept coming to the clinic, many of the terrible and often desperate concerns she expressed were supplanted by a theme which became the major issue in treatment, as it was in her life. This was her long-standing bitter quarrel with her mother. It was somehow linked to what seemed an almost irresistible need on Phyllis' part to return to her mother's home each weekend. She had no idea why she kept going back, particularly since she always seemed to have such a terrible time. In fact, she usually found herself drinking, even drunk, before arriving home. And she frequently stayed drunk most of the weekend.

Over the months we worked on this theme of Phyllis' need to return to mother, and over the months her anger towards her mother grew. I had seldom heard such venomous hatred as that which wracked her after her weekends at home. And it was almost as if the more she hated the more she needed to return. But why?

As we talked it became clearer. Going home was a way of reassuring herself that she had not hurt her mother by what she said about her in treatment; but it was more than that. When she allowed her mother to humiliate and degrade her, she assured herself not only that she had not hurt her

mother, but that she could not hurt her. By going home, and
getting drunk, and sleeping with men, she was in effect saying,
"See, I'm not really defying you by running off to New York.
I'm not trying to set myself over you. I'm really just like you
in every miserable, bad way."

As she reached this understanding Phyllis became calm,
even radiant. She announced that she had decided to be nice
to herself for a change, and she looked it. She was wearing
an attractive new dress, and a new coat and lipstick that set
off her beautiful blue eyes. Her unruly hair was set in the
first permanent wave she had ever had. She was through with
the penitent trips home, she reported, and had told her mother
that she would not be back the following weekend, or for
the Thanksgiving holidays the week after that. She did not
seem elated. But she had started a diet and lost nine pounds
in a week . . .

This good fortune did not last long. Phyllis called the
following week to say that she could not keep her appointment.
Later I learned what had happened. Things had continued
to go wonderfully well for the six days after her last visit
to the clinic. Then on the morning of her next visit she had
awakened in a panic after a vivid, terrifying dream:

"I am back in my home town in a telephone booth,
and I am about to have a baby. My father and brother came,
and I have the baby. It is very realistic, pains and everything.
The cord is there, and I don't know what to do with it. My
father kneels down and begins gnawing on it like a rat. It
hurts. I am very frightened and start screaming. Then he bites
through it. I woke up terrified."

Phyllis said that she knew that the dream was about
". . . my fear of leaving home. The umbilical cord is what
binds me to my parents. I am terribly afraid of having it
cut."

She had bounded out of bed after the dream, shaking,
jittery, tense. The feelings mounted to unbearable anxiety.
When she began to shake all over, she found herself debating
whether this was a shaking chill which meant that she had
pneumonia, or whether it was simply fear, in which case she

was surely going insane. She decided on pneumonia: "It was serious and physical, and would explain why I felt so awful." Leaving her apartment early in the morning, she rushed home.

Phyllis greeted her astonished mother with the report that she was deathly ill and in desperate need of help. "And just as soon as I was there, I felt much better. I just went to bed and let Mother feed me, and I ate and ate and ate." By the end of the week she had regained the nine pounds, and her anxiety was decreasing.

The following week, having bolstered her courage with "a few drinks," Phyllis left home to keep her appointment with me. Glumly she told me what had happened. She spoke about being afraid of me and afraid of coming in to see me. "We have talked a lot about my hatred for my mother, but we've neglected my need for her. We just ignored that, and I need her terribly." I agreed.

For a month she continued to be tense and frightened during the day, and drunk at night. The old feeling that people were watching her returned with unprecedented severity. As we were walking into the office, she looked around her in such a frightened, trapped way that I asked if she were afraid of being in the office. She said that she was, but it wasn't just my office; she looked around her this way all the time now. She told me of spending every free hour at home with her mother. Usually she felt better there, and she complained that she couldn't understand why. "The price of going back is my self-respect. You can't have any idea of how bad it is there, everyone yelling all the time, Mother heckling me for everything I do. Someone is always yelling, 'Do this, do that' . . . 'I'll break your arm if you don't stop that' . . . 'I'll knock your teeth out if you don't do that!' "

As the months went by, however, Phyllis became less frightened. She no longer felt that people were watching her, and she no longer gave the impression of feeling trapped when she was in my office. On the other hand, she became increasingly morose and sad. Her communications were sparse and hostile. For long periods she would sit silently, responding to my questions and comments solely with gestures, or not at all. Then she began to break her appointments, and I found it harder and harder to keep track of what was happening in her life. Clearly she was drinking heavily, and borrowing to pay for it. Her alcoholism was interfering with her work, her friendships, her treatment, and ultimately, her life.

One morning I was awakened by the telephone ringing, to hear a weak voice saying, "I've slashed my wrists." In fact she had, but the bleeding had stopped by the time I reached her, and she bitterly handed me her blood-caked suicide note. It read in part: "I've got to be punished because I am a monster inside, all ugly and creepy, and I'll never be any different." She had carried out part of the punishment she felt she needed by cutting a deep "H" into her arm, "... to brand myself as a homosexual." Now exhausted, all tension and anxiety gone, she just wanted to go to bed and rest.

This crisis passed, as had others. But both of us realized that what we were doing was not enough. Ten months after her last ill-fated attempt at dieting, with treatment at a standstill and her life going downhill, Phyllis entered a mental hospital.

Its doctors took complete care of her, and I saw Phyllis only infrequently when I went as a visitor. But these visits, and talks with her psychiatrist, gave me a good picture of her course in the hospital. The treatment program helped her a great deal. She took part in a wide variety of hospital activities. When she left the hospital after ten months, she was considerably improved. During her hospital stay, she also had gone on a diet.

This diet is worthy of note. She began it soon after her admission, when she was still quite depressed; she continued it until her discharge. And she lost more weight than during any of her previous diets, 80 pounds. She weighed 275 on admission and 195 at discharge. How did this weight loss affect her emotionally? It did not have the devastating consequences of her earlier ones. She did not undergo another period of panic and disorganization like the one that had marked the onset of her illness in our clinic. In fact, she became much less depressed.

What conclusion did I draw from this experience at dieting? For one, Phyllis was able for the first time in her life to lose a large amount of weight without becoming depressed. It seems reasonable to believe that this favorable outcome was due to the active treatment and support she received in the hospital. She was anxious and tense during this time, but no more so than usual.

In my mind I began to separate the ill effects from dieting into two categories: psychological and biological. For Phyllis, Mrs. Rosselini, and Mrs. Malone, psychological factors seemed to play a central role in their dieting depressions. Dieting and weight loss, the symbols of freedom and independence, and the subsequent difficulties of living with this freedom, were too prominent to ignore. But biological factors, the effects of food deprivation, may well have increased their vulnerability to the psychological conflicts. Certainly non-specific results of weight reduction, such as irritability and tension, could affect the obese as well as the non-obese.

I treated Phyllis for two years after her discharge from the hospital, until I moved away from New York. And I kept in touch with her for several years after that. The most important development in her life was to join Alcoholics Anonymous. When I last heard from her, she had been sober for eight years. Her performance at work had improved as soon as she stopped drinking, and she gradually rose to a responsible position in a large company. After considerable sexual experimentation with men and women, and much associated turmoil, she had accepted her homosexuality and had been living relatively happily with another woman for some years. She had been able to keep her weight below 200 pounds. And she had achieved a dearly won sense of pride, and an ability to manage her life.

At this time very little had appeared in the medical literature about the complications of losing weight. Yet concern with obesity and weight reduction had been mounting until it had assumed the proportions of a national neurosis. The time seemed ripe for a report on the problem.

The first part of my report dealt with the frequency of

emotional disturbances during efforts at weight reduction. Among the vulnerable persons I had treated, nine of the first twenty-five had become disturbed while dieting. Four of these disturbances had occurred while I was treating them; eight others had occurred previously. (Three of the patients experienced two illnesses each, making a total of twelve illnesses in nine patients.)

The next part of the report described the illnesses themselves. They all had two distinct phases, characterized first by symptoms of anxiety, and later by those of depression. In addition, half the illnesses had been initiated by a period of mild elation, with some overactivity and increased feelings of well-being. The elation would begin at about the time the patient decided to break off an important dependency relationship, and was often first manifested by the feelings of exultation with which the patient celebrated his or her apparent freedom. These feelings were intensified by the decision to diet. Many of the patients had long cherished secret dreams of the extravagant benefits to be achieved by weight reduction, and when, after years of indecision, they sought to live out this fantasy, it was with excited anticipation. This heightened mood persisted for weeks and even months.

Typically the elation was abruptly terminated by a short period of anxiety. Some apparently minor incident would bring home to the patients the consequences of the course they were following, and they would react with severe anxiety. During this time they would become preoccupied with the danger of living without the support they had so gratuitously cut off. And perhaps more importantly, the patients would begin to fear the retaliation of the authority they had defied.

Within a week or two anxiety would be displaced by a depressive reaction that might last for months. During this period the patients would feel generally depressed, with frequent crying spells and disturbed sleep. In each case the disorder was severe enough to interfere with the ability to work. Suicidal ruminations were common, but self-destructive attempts were rare.

Recovery occurred in all the patients after illnesses which

lasted from six weeks to a year, but the factors leading to recovery were not clear. Although all the patients discontinued their reducing diets soon after the onset of severe symptoms, increased food intake did not terminate the illnesses. Furthermore, in each case the disrupted personal relationship was restored, but this could as easily have been a result of the recovery as a cause.

The report on the 25 patients was now complete. But they were a select group. Referred to us because of the severity of their obesity or difficulty in its management, they undoubtedly represented a high proportion of emotionally disturbed people. I didn't know whether this proportion was higher in this particular group than in the average severely obese group. The usefulness of the report to the practicing physician would be greatly increased if, in addition to providing information about these more difficult patients, I could say something about dieting by the average obese patient who comes to the family doctor. Specifically, how often do these patients develop such symptoms when they diet?

The nearest thing to a cross-section of dieters was the group of patients who came to the Nutrition Clinic of the New York Hospital. I had become well acquainted with this Clinic in the course of referring patients for reducing diets. It was an ideal place to study the average overweight dieter, for it treated a true cross-section of them. I was able to arrange for interviews of 100 patients.

Instead of trying to keep in touch with all 100 patients to find out how they tolerated their *present* reducing diets, we simply asked them about their *previous* diets. This method had the disadvantage of requiring patients to remember events that might be long forgotten. It was subject to the well-known retrospective falsification which can occur in such recall. Nevertheless, it allowed us to obtain information on 100 percent of our group of patients, an unusual record in the study of obese people. Furthermore, the process was very economical.

We were surprised by the results. 72 of the 100 patients had dieted previously, several of them on many occasions. Of these, 54 percent reported such symptoms as nervousness, weakness and irritability during at least one reducing regimen; and 55 percent of all such regimens were characterized by the presence of symptoms.

The report of this study on "The Dieting Depression" was greeted with interest by many physicians. I was pleased by this interest because of the possibility that it might herald a change in their usual harsh attitudes toward such patients. Perhaps it might lead them to treat them with more respect. As early as medical school I had been aware of the condescending and punitive attitude of some doctors towards their obese patients. Even physicians who were relatively uncritical of them still found them frustrating, boring, irritating.

As my teaching had put me in contact with more and more practitioners, I had begun to sense that their negative attitudes were the result of two underlying assumptions: first, that weight reduction programs are effective, and second, that they are harmless. Compared with the more acute diseases with which physicians dealt, obesity seemed a trivial disorder. If, in addition, they thought that weight reduction was an easy matter, they might quite understandably be frustrated by the failure of their patients to lose weight.

By this time my own experience had convinced me that weight-reduction programs were not nearly as effective as was generally believed. And the "Dieting Depression" study indicated that they might not be harmless. To my great satisfaction, physicians on the firing line seemed ready to accept both these points. If their treatment of obese patients produced results no worse than those of others, they had no reason to blame themselves or to criticize their patients. And the idea that a treatment might have adverse side reactions was a well-recognized part of medical practice. The demonstration that treatment for obesity could produce such ill effects tended to legitimize the treatment *and* the condition toward which treatment was directed. As a result physicians were increasingly able to see obesity as a respectable medical problem and less as a sign of moral weakness. Respecting their patients' problem made it easier to respect the patients themselves.

At times, however, I became concerned by an overly

enthusiastic endorsement of the idea that weight reduction might have its hazards for obese people. For it could be used to discourage any treatment of obesity. Such an attitude was particularly distressing because evidence was accumulating that weight reduction could have some very favorable effects upon health.

One particularly significant study cited people who had been refused life insurance because of obesity. They had then lost weight and consequently qualified for life insurance. These people showed far lower mortality rates than did obese people. For the women in the study the mortality rate was as low as if they had never been obese. These findings made it a singularly inappropriate time to discourage all efforts at weight reduction; and I was concerned that our study was being used to support this negative point of view.

In the years following publication of "The Dieting Depression" many papers were published on the subject. Some supported the view that there was little if any correlation between depression and dieting; others supported my less optimistic conclusions. Controversy grew as to whether dieting made obese people feel better or worse. I became confused, and I had to assume that others must be at least as confused. How was the physician in practice to interpret these conflicting reports?

It was not until I sat down to write this book that I was finally able to resolve this conflict to my own satisfaction. For once I had the leisure to review the literature, it became apparent that most forms of dieting carried with them a high likelihood of emotional disturbance. And, paradoxically, the strongest evidence in support of this conclusion was provided by precisely those reports which denied the dangers of dieting. One, for example, reported symptoms in half the people undertaking reducing diets; another reported premature discontinuation by 75 percent. These dismal figures applied not only to the more lenient diets of people living at home, but even to the carefully supervised long-term diets in hospitals.

And there, for the time being, the matter of dieting and depression rests. It has left us with respect for the difficulties of dieting, and that is to the good. Obese people need all the understanding they can get. And it has not precluded efforts at weight reduction by those people who must lose weight for medical, as opposed to cosmetic, reasons. Finally, it has given us a baseline against which to measure new methods of treatment for obesity. If a new treatment is as effective as, or more effective than, the old ones, and if it does not produce as much emotional difficulty, clearly it has much to recommend it. And such a treatment may well be at hand, as we shall see in Chapter 8.

three
Binge-Eating

An invitation to give a talk at a psychiatric hospital in New York stimulated my next endeavor—an inquiry which defined a second eating pattern, the eating binge. This inquiry did not start from observations about patients, as had the study of night eating, but rather from new information about brain mechanisms, derived from experiments with animals. The discovery of brain areas which control eating was still fresh, and we had not yet fully assimilated the unexpected finding that there were not one but two pairs of such areas. One triggers eating and the other inhibits it. Why this division of labor?

The idea that there are brain areas that stimulate eating was not surprising; such areas had been postulated long before

49

their discovery. What was a surprise was the discovery of satiety areas which inhibit eating. For traditionally, satiety had been viewed as a purely incidental aspect of eating—what happened when the drive to eat ran out of steam. But if that were all there is to satiety, separate brain areas to inhibit eating would be quite unnecessary. Yet satiety areas existed, and their destruction was followed promptly by over-eating and obesity. Furthermore, the over-eating which followed destruction of the satiety areas had some strange and unexpected characteristics.

For example, if rats with their satiety areas destroyed were allowed free access to food, they over-ate in an uncontrolled manner, often consuming twice their usual amount of food, as if all the brakes had been removed. But when any obstruction was placed in their way, their food intake fell not only below its usual level, but even below that of non-obese rats faced with a similar obstruction. It made no difference what form the obstruction took, whether it involved lifting heavy covers to reach the food, solving mazes, pressing levers, electric shocks, even adulteration with quinine. Faced with such impediments, the obese rats simply sat down on the job and ate *less* than non-obese rats under the same circumstances.

This research exploded traditional views of "hunger" as a unitary phenomenon. Hunger as defined by how much food an animal eats is apparently quite different from hunger as defined by how hard the animal will work to obtain food.

These experiments with animals also had a liberating effect upon our understanding of the way obese people eat. We were no longer forced to account for all over-eating in terms of increased hunger (although that could, of course, still be the case). We now knew that over-eating might also result from decreased satiety, and that these two forms of over-eating might well differ dramatically.

The night-eating pattern seemed a classic instance of over-eating as a failure of satiety—for a characteristic complaint of night-eaters was an inability to stop eating once they started. They rarely spoke of being hungry. Instead, I heard

time and again how difficult it was to stop eating as long
as food was available, how they found themselves nibbling
and just could not seem to stop. Yet if food were not available,
they rarely developed any strong desire to eat or made any
great effort to obtain food. Even when severely agitated, they
would rarely so much as leave the house to buy food.

So much for over-eating due to failure of satiety. What
about over-eating due to an increased hunger drive? Did it
occur in humans as well as in experimental animals? The
question kept coming back more and more insistently. So I
set about searching for obese people who described their over-
eating in terms suggestive of increased hunger. I soon met
a promising candidate.

Hyman Cohen was a 37-year-old high school teacher
referred to me by a mutual friend. This friend said that Mr.
Cohen was a "compulsive eater," and his description of this
eating made it sound as if it might be due to an increased
hunger drive. The description intrigued me. So did another
aspect: the possibility of intensive treatment of an obese man.
I had already come to realize how infrequently men seek
treatment for their obesity. Of the 25 obese patients who served
as subjects for the night-eating study, only two were men.
And I knew neither well.

From the moment that Hyman Cohen walked through
the door, it was clear that he was quite different from the
passive, obese women with whom I had grown so familiar.
A big, burly man with large shoulders and a massive chest,
he strode into the office, rolling as the very obese must because
of the thickness of their thighs. And the girth of his upper
arms forced his arms out from his sides, something in the
manner of a wrestler. He was clearly obese—carrying 272
pounds on his five-foot-nine frame—but the impression that
he gave was not what I had come to expect from my experiences with obese women. He had tremendous vitality and
vigor.

Mr. Cohen shook my hand with a bone-crunching grasp;
later I learned that he spent a great deal of time in weight-lift-
ing and body building exercises. Even when he sat down,

uncomfortably bulging out of the chair and bursting out of his clothing, he still seemed forceful and aggressive. His face was round and full, his eyes slits behind large horn-rimmed glasses, his head covered with short, brown, curly hair. He began speaking at once and continued at length, almost without interruption. His speech was booming and forceful. He punctuated his remarks with frequent outbursts of laughter, at first nervous and shy, but eventually loud and even raucous. At times he spoke of what he called his "Rabelaisian" activities—and it seemed to me, as I sat listening silently to his flood of speech, that Rabelaisian was a fitting description of his entire appearance and manner.

Mr. Cohen got to the point at once. The immediate stimulus for his coming to see me was that he was being considered for the position of principal at the high school where he taught. He wanted the job because it meant a substantial salary increase. But he now weighed over 270 pounds and could not pass the required physical examination. He had six months to reduce, and if he were successful, he was certain that he would not only pass the physical but get the job.

"So, I want you to peel this weight off and get me down to fighting shape."

Mr. Cohen went on to say that he had a problem with biting his fingernails and held up his hands to show nails bitten to the quick, pink, tender skin bulging out about them, and traces of what appeared to be clotted blood in the depressions at the bottom of the nails. He also reported that he was always in debt. He thought his indebtedness, his nail-biting, and his obesity were somehow connected, but he was not sure how.

He beamed proudly as he told me of this connection and went on to say that he knew a great deal about himself. He had been, he explained, "psychoanalyzed" four or five years before. It developed that he had seen a psychoanalyst for treatment at that time, going twice a week for about a year. He said that it had been a resounding success, that it had cleared up all of his emotional problems and had left him with deep insights, not only into himself but also into those around him.

He counted his "psychoanalysis" as one of the most important experiences in his life, if not *the* most important. Although he had not had any serious emotional problems before the treatment, it had, he said, left him in a state of perfect contentment. He went on to describe his happy marriage, his lovely son, his challenging job. I had become accustomed to hearing obese people tell me in our first interview how well their lives were going. But I had never encountered a tale of such utter bliss.

Finally, about forty minutes after he entered the office, Mr. Cohen began to run down a bit. I was then able to put into words my mounting doubts. "If things are going so well," I asked, "why are you coming to see me?"

Brought up sharply, Mr. Cohen paused and looked quizzically at me. "For psychotherapy, of course."

I admitted my bewilderment. "Why?"

Mr. Cohen replied in a tone of voice that implied any damn fool ought to know the answer to that one: "Well, obesity *is* a psychosomatic problem, isn't it?"

I hesitated. Despite the countless things he had already told me about himself, I had the feeling that I did not know this man at all. And I was increasingly puzzled about what it was he wanted of me. Finally I began slowly: "Yes . . . People do consider obesity a psychosomatic disease . . . But it must have a number of different causes. . . ." I floundered along, discomfited by his growing and very apparent disappointment.

For a time neither of us said anything. Then I tried again. "Well, what puzzles me is, your life seems to be going along very well. You haven't told me about any problems. . . ."

"Just the obesity. That's right. I don't have any problems except for the obesity. That's what I'm here for, to get it cleared up."

"But you say that you don't have any problems, no worries or conflicts that might be causing the obesity . . ." I ventured.

"That's right," he replied. "Emotions are definitely not involved. There is no connection there. I haven't had any emotional problems since my psychoanalysis."

"Well, then, why . . ." I began, and then I stopped. Our time was up, and I welcomed relief from this perplexing encounter. Perhaps we could do better next time. I told Mr. Cohen I did not feel I had yet gotten a grasp on the problem. Would he like to come back next week at the same time?

"I certainly would, doctor, I'll be here. You can count on that." He rose, crushed my hand with his vise-like grasp, and strode out the door.

I approached our next meeting with concern. What was it Mr. Cohen really wanted? How could I clarify it? What could I do about whatever it was that was bothering him? How was I to begin?

I needn't have worried. Mr. Cohen was waiting for me when I arrived at the office, strode in and seated himself with assurance and asked, "Well, doctor, where do we go from here? I feel that I want to do whatever I can to be a good experimental subject. I want to help your research in every possible way."

"Experimental subject?" I asked.

"Yes," he went on. "I've had a long talk with Mr. Leibowitz (the mutual friend who had referred him to me) about your research, and I want to do everything within my power to help it along."

I murmured feebly that I did not want him to think of himself as an experimental subject, that I considered our relationship as one of patient and doctor, and that I saw my job as trying to help him decide what difficulties he was having and what he might do about them. Not surprisingly, in view of my failure in that attempt during our last visit, Mr. Cohen appeared a bit crestfallen. "Don't you want to see me any more?" he pleaded.

Gamely trying to preserve the illusion that I was exploring the possibility of psychotherapy with him, I returned to our discussion of the previous week and said that I didn't think we had gotten clear on his problem.

He immediately assured me, "The problem is my obesity, and what the hell I am going to do about it. It's completely out of control. I've gained nearly 60 pounds in the last year and I'm eating all the time now. I've had this crazy idea '. . . Dr. Stunkard is going to take care of me. So I can do anything I want to, because when I get to him everything will be all right.' " He stopped and looked imploringly at me. "You've just got to help me."

Suddenly it all became clear. Beneath the bluster and bravado was a frightened man, desperately appealing for help. How could I have failed to see this?

The next step was easy. "O.K. How do we do it?"

"Well, as I see it," he began, his confidence returning, "it's all just a matter of will power. I can start a diet any time I want to. And I can lose a hell of a lot of weight when I am on one. But right now my will power just doesn't seem to be up to it. That's where you come in. It's like hiring a policeman to check on me. If I am going to have to face the scales each week, I am simply going to have to stop eating so much. It's as simple as that.

"Also it's a little like being a Catholic and going to confession. When I was going to see my analyst, I would confess my sins and then I would feel better. I got some release last week just telling you about my eating. I never talk to anyone else about it. It makes me think of *Crime and Punishment,* like the criminal who always has to talk about his crimes. There's another book about it, *Island in the Sun.* It has the same theme—the criminal with an implacable desire to tell of his crimes . . . to confess his sins."

Warming to the topic, he went on. Finally I said that I was impressed with the way he described himself as a criminal—as guilty of some crime because of his eating.

"Of course. This damned weight is not only damaging my job prospects but it's shortening my life expectancy. So, indirectly, it's going to hurt my wife as well as me."

I said that his talk sounded much more urgent than concern over job prospects and life expectancy. These seemed relatively abstract long-range considerations. He seemed, I insisted, to be talking about something much more urgent. What was it?

"My guilt drives me here," he said. "But why do I feel so guilty? Why is it so out of proportion to what I have done? It's not that terrible to over-eat and yet I feel it is."

"Do you have any idea why it seems so terrible?" I asked.

"I just don't know. I just don't have any idea. It's just that this eating has become an obsession with me. I think about it all the time. It's the first thing I think of when I wake up in the morning and it's the last thing I think of when I go to bed at night." As Mr. Cohen talked on, he kept referring to his eating. Food kept coming into the conversation with a persistence that amazed me. Almost everything he talked about had to do with food. I had never heard anything like it.

He told of a time when he had thought that his eating might be an attempt to obtain gratification that he was not receiving in other spheres. For example, when he was younger, for a long time he had wanted to have a car and had not been able to afford it. "It was like having a car was a kind of gratification. I thought maybe my eating was trying to get the gratification that I wanted from having a car. So I thought that if I bought a car I might be able to lose weight. In those days I wanted a car so badly *that I could taste it.* But of course when I got the car, it didn't help.

"All these things are just rationalizations for why I really eat. They're excuses . . . They fool me. It's like a battle between me as an individual and my appetite. I try tricks and sometimes I can fool my appetite, and then it turns right around and tricks me."

Much of what Mr. Cohen told me in those early days was formulated in terms of "victories" and "defeats," or of instances of when "I was good" or "I was bad." The "victories," when he was "good," invariably involved instances of resisting the temptation to eat, reminiscences about experiences on diets, accounts of amounts of weight, often very large, that he had lost during earlier attempts at dieting. Conversely, "defeats" and "being bad" were instances of succumbing to the temptation to eat, of breaking a diet, of going to some absurd length to "prevent anyone from witnessing the shameful act I was just about to perform.

"Just yesterday, for example, I did a thing that makes no sense at all. I knew my wife had left something to eat in a closet in the kitchen. I kept thinking about it all the time, couldn't get it out of my mind. Then when she went to take a bath, I slipped in and stole it and ate it. Then I suddenly realized that naturally she would notice that it was gone when she looked in the closet again. So all of my elaborate precautions to avoid being discovered were pointless. Why do I do things like that?"

I shrugged my shoulders, "What kind of food was it?"

He frowned. "You know, I can't remember.

"I am a sleepwalker, too, you know," he volunteered. "My wife says that I do it every night sometimes. Usually I'm terribly angry. I'm shouting about somebody and I'm mad at them. It's always a man, 'George' or 'Dick' or something like that. I don't know who. And I eat then too. My wife says that I act in a very rational way. I get up, go to the icebox, get out food and eat it. And I have absolutely no memory of it the next morning. What do you think of that, Doc?"

Even his dreams reflected his concern with eating. "In this one dream this neighbor lady of ours was at dinner with my wife and me, and we were all eating roast stuffed veal. That's one of my favorite foods. Then, later, I was walking on the Lower East Side and I was gnawing a large, greasy piece of veal I had picked out of a garbage can. People were standing there watching me make a spectacle of myself, and I felt terribly ashamed of how I must look. But there wasn't anything I could do about it. Then that same night I had another dream. My fingernails were bitten to the quick. They were bleeding and I was sucking the blood. I felt miserable."

I suggested that we try to learn more about the circumstances under which his over-eating took place. It was clear that although he often ate at night, he was not suffering from the night-eating pattern. But perhaps his over-eating followed

some pattern. I suggested that he pay particular attention
to the times when he over-ate most heavily, and that we try
to see if we could find any pattern in these occasions.

He applied himself diligently to the task, but at first
without success. He seemed to eat in a chaotic manner
throughout the day. Almost any kind of frustration, or
achievement, could trigger his eating. Nevertheless, he began
to feel better, the intense pressure to eat slackened, and he
began to lose weight. It was under these circumstances, six
weeks after he entered treatment, that he described the events
which led me to recognize a second eating pattern.

The appointment began with a long pause. Then Mr.
Cohen said, "I suppose you noticed the weight gain."

I nodded. His weight, which had fallen to 265 pounds
in the previous six weeks, was again 272 pounds.

He started to talk two or three times, but could not.
He looked up at the ceiling and then towards the door in
an agony of embarrassment. Finally, he took a deep breath
and said, "Well, I have to begin some time."

He began to talk about New Year's Day, two days before.
He had told his wife that he was going down town to his
chess club. While on the highway he began to think of going
over to Newark to see a burlesque show. "So I did it. Just
like that. As soon as the idea came into my mind I just went
ahead and went over to Minsky's . . . Naturally I couldn't
tell my wife about it . . . I hadn't seen a burlesque show
in years. It was like when I was young."

Puzzled, I asked about his eating.

"No problem with eating. I kept it under 1000 calories,"
he said.

"Well, then, the weight . . . ?" I asked.

"That was the next day. I got my check cashed. I usually
eat to celebrate the occasion. I don't have any idea why. So
I knew it might happen. On the way to the bank I steeled
myself. I kept reminding myself of the treatment and about
my New Year's resolution about dieting and about having
to face you and the scales."

He continued, slowing down to a less frantic pace. "Then I got the check cashed. And I kept out a hundred dollars. And everything just seemed to go blank. I don't know what happened. All of my good intentions just seemed to fade away. They just didn't seem to mean anything any more. I just said, 'What the hell,' and I started eating, and what I did then was an absolute sin."

He detailed what he had eaten. It was a tremendous amount and he had gained eight pounds during that one day. He had started in a grocery store, where he had bought a cake, pieces of pie and cookies, and he told of driving through the heavy midtown traffic with one hand, while pulling food out of the bag and eating it with the other.

After consuming all his grocery purchases as rapidly as possible, he had set out on a furtive round of the local restaurants, staying only a short time in each and eating only a small amount. Constantly in dread of discovery, he was not at all sure what "sin" he felt he was committing. He only knew that it wasn't pleasurable. "I didn't enjoy it at all. It just happened. It's like part of me blacked out, just wasn't there any more. And when that happened there was nothing there except the food and me—all alone."

Finally, he went into a delicatessen, bought another twenty dollars worth of food and drove home, eating all the way, "until my gut ached from all that I had eaten.

"My wife knew what I was doing, but she knows enough not to make an issue of it. Only later, in the evening, she seemed kind of wistful and asked me, 'When are you going to see Dr. Stunkard again?' "

Mr. Cohen sat looking ahead, a deep frown wrinkling his forehead. "And that's the whole truth, your honor."

I asked him how he felt, and he replied. "I feel some relief from telling you all this. I don't know why. Maybe it was like when I was seeing my analyst. I remember telling him about an eating binge. I had been walking down the street with nothing at all on my mind and looked across and saw a grocery store. The next thing I knew I was in the store

buying food. It was uncanny. It frightened me, not remembering how I had gotten there. But once I got started, there
wasn't a thing I could do about it. I remember that time
I spent $25 on groceries, and I had them in a big basket
and I hired a taxi and was riding all over New York eating
up a storm, eating away until my gut ached." He began to
laugh as he told of this earlier "binge," and he went on roaring
with laughter as he told of the long taxi ride which ended
at his home with a half-empty basket of food.

The memory of that earlier "binge," and of discussing
it with his analyst, persisted. "I had a very significant dream
that time," he said, and went on to describe quite vividly
a dream which must have occurred at least four years before.

"I was in a subway, on the Broadway-Seventh Avenue
line just after it comes out of the ground. The car was filled
with nude girls who were skipping rope. I wanted them to
let me in on the fun, but they excluded me. I was very sad
when I woke up."

Mr. Cohen said that he remembered that when he had
awakened from this dream he felt that it had been very
significant, and could hardly wait to tell his analyst. "It was
like he would be able to tell me what my problem was, and
then everything would be solved. Sort of like magic. And my
analyst was great. He told me, 'That's easy. That dream is
about *Man on a Tightrope.*' That was a book I had just read
and we had been talking about. It was about a man who
was unfaithful to his wife."

I asked what the analyst had meant, and Mr. Cohen
said, "I don't know except that I was having trouble with
my wife at that time. My analyst never said much, but that
was what he was talking about, about the trouble with my
wife. It reminded me of a quotation from Oscar Wilde: 'Most
men would be unfaithful to their wives if they weren't so
lazy.' That's the way I am. I've never been unfaithful, but
I would be, without any compunction, if the opportunity arose.
But I won't go looking."

Mr. Cohen's comments kept coming back towards his
wife. I thought of his trip to the burlesque show the day before

the binge, how he had introduced the topic of his weight gain by talking about that trip, and how he had taken it for granted that he could not tell his wife about it. I suggested that he tell me more about what had happened that day.

Mr. Cohen said that he wasn't at all sure how this was related to his eating, but he would be glad to talk about it. "There was a party at the neighbors' and everyone had been talking about pornography. I'm interested in pornography, and I was very interested when they talked about going to a burlesque show. But my wife didn't like it at all. She said that she thought it was all pretty disgusting. So I found myself saying the same thing too, that it was pretty disgusting. But I really would have liked to go, and if my wife had said she wanted to, I would have. Then some of the neighbors invited some of the people who had been at the party to see pornographic movies they had rented, and they didn't ask me. I felt terribly left out. I felt that if I hadn't talked like such a prude at the party they would have asked me to see the pornographic movies. That just stuck in my mind. That was what I was thinking about when I decided to go over to Minsky's. I don't know why it was so important to me."

This account of Mr. Cohen's marked a turning point in my understanding. Until then I had been overwhelmed, as had he, by what seemed a chaotic, patternless quality to his over-eating. But his talk of "an eating binge" had caught my attention. Although these binges might occur at night, their form was clearly quite different from the night-eating pattern. Here, it seemed, was a distinctive behavior; it might be possible to characterize it as fully as the night-eating pattern. Eagerly I set about this task, and, caught up by my enthusiasm, Mr. Cohen also threw himself into it.

First, what did it feel like when he was over-eating?

"There are two things I notice when I am eating like that. First of all, I just love the feeling of swallowing. I have my mouth full of food and I'm gulping it down, hardly even bothering to chew it, just stuffing it down. Then there's the feeling in my stomach, a full feeling, a very full feeling. It gets so full that it's painful, and I think that that's one of the things I'm looking for in a binge—eating so damned much that my gut aches. When that happens, then I can usually call off the binge, and a damned good thing, too. I might split my stomach wide open with all that I eat.

"Then, often I'll be drinking during a binge. I'll have a craving for spicy foods and this will make me thirsty, and so I'll drink beer. I might polish off six or eight bottles of beer just to keep me going, and then I'll want more food."

And how did he feel during these binges?

"Well," he began slowly, "I wonder. Sometimes I think maybe it's fun to be eating that way. But I don't know. I don't think it's fun. I usually feel pretty bad while I'm eating. I don't feel I'm in control any more. It's like I'm being driven to it."

And how did he feel after the binge? What was it like then?

"Well, there's this ache in my gut, and sometimes it gets pretty bad. It used to get bad enough that I would make myself vomit, to get all that stuff out of there. I'd forgotten about that. I used to do it quite a lot before my analysis, but I haven't done it at all since then. I guess the analysis cured me of it. But I remember now how I would make myself vomit, and then go back and start eating all over again."

"And what then?" I asked.

"I'd just feel like hell. I'd feel that I should be punished for my sins." He smiled in embarrassment. "There should be some retribution for the shameful act that I had performed."

I don't remember Mr. Cohen ever saying that he felt like a murderer in the aftermath of an eating binge, but I was to hear others talk this way. When I commented about the images he used to describe himself after a binge, saying that he seemed to feel like a criminal, he replied, as if it were the most obvious thing in the world, "of course."

As I thought about this exaggerated feeling of guilt, it occurred to me that I didn't remember Mr. Cohen ever having expressed guilt about anything else in his life. Had he felt so guilty about things other than eating? The answer was "no."

I briefly entertained the notion that his strong sense of guilt might have prevented any kind of activity that would make him feel guilty. But this supposition seemed unlikely on the face of it. He was an unusually energetic man, and I already knew that his Rabelaisian tastes extended far beyond eating. Indeed, as treatment continued, and as he came to trust me, he unfolded tales of activities that were antisocial, sometimes criminal. Far from being guilt-ridden, he experienced no qualms about any of them.

Even in early childhood he had stolen money from the cash register of his parents' store. There was a long history of cheating on his income tax and of passing bad checks. He consistently stole books from the library and pilfered small items from drugstores. His reckless driving resulted in a stream of traffic violations.

"I'm really a very amoral person," he observed. "But I don't feel guilty about anything except eating. Last term I stole a purse from one of the teachers at my school and made off with the $40 in it. She had left it in my office and forgotten it. At first I wasn't planning to steal it. I just hid it, planning to play a joke on her. But then later she told me she thought someone had taken it from her office. I realized she would never suspect me. So I took the money out and then took the purse home and burned it."

There was just one time that I remember Mr. Cohen saying he felt guilty over stealing. He described an episode at the house of a boy he was tutoring, while he was alone in the living room waiting for the boy to appear. "There was a big box of candy there and I started to eat it. I got a piece of sticky candy, and while I was chewing it, a filling came out. It was just terrible. 'Now I'll have to have a big dental job and it's going to cost me a lot of money.' " His shoulders slumped. He looked contrite. And when he spoke it was in a low, despairing tone, *"Things like that could ruin me."*

The guilt after an eating binge had one striking consequence. It often drove Mr. Cohen to diet. Many things could start him dieting—it might be something as trivial as having gotten through the day with little food. But the diets that followed binges had a special desperate quality to them. This was true of the first diet he undertook after he started treatment. It was about four months after he first came to see me, and followed the trip to Minsky's burlesque and his subsequent binge.

He began the diet with a terrible urgency. "I am an extremist. I just have to get on a strict diet and get this weight off, come hell or high water." As had often happened with such guilt-inspired diets, he ate very little and lost weight rapidly. He was soon commenting, "Once I really get into a diet it gets easier, and I find it less and less difficult to avoid food." Everything seemed to favor the diet. "I think my stomach must have shrunk. This morning I went into the place where I usually have breakfast and ordered black coffee, and when they brought me the coffee, they also brought me a bagel, which I usually eat with it. I just looked at the bagel and it revolted me. It was actual physical revulsion," he explained proudly. "Now I know I am on my way."

Such success in dieting was accompanied this time, as on other, similar occasions, by exuberance and a heightened mood. "It's like magic . . . I can control myself with ease. There just isn't a struggle any more. Things that would have thrown me before now just slide off my back without a second thought. I've even got my wife convinced. You remember how she used to feel about my coming here? Well, now she says she *believes* in psychiatry.

"The funny thing is, Doctor, that even hunger pangs feel good. They are really pleasurable; they make me feel as if I'm accomplishing something."

But these accomplishments were not to last. Hyman Cohen himself noted the fatal flaw. "The trouble with being an extremist," he observed, "is that it works the other way too. If I don't diet perfectly, I just give up. I say 'Oh hell, what's the use?' And then everything goes to hell and I just eat or drink. I might drink four quarts of beer, or a fifth of whiskey, and eat until my gut aches."

A month after starting the diet, and 25 pounds lighter, Mr. Cohen failed to diet perfectly and promptly gave up. It was a sequence he had repeated 20 times before. This time,

however, there was a difference which made a profound impression upon Mr. Cohen, and intrigued and puzzled me.
He stopped biting his fingernails for the first time in his life,
and he never started again.

The vividness with which this highly intelligent man
described events taught me a great deal about the distinctive
pattern he called, appropriately enough, an "eating binge."
My later experience with other patients confirmed much of
what Mr. Cohen had taught me about this kind of over-eating:
the sudden, out-of-the-blue way it came on, its orgiastic quality, the feeling of loss of control, and the compulsion to eat
until the stomach was full, even painful.

There was also a pattern to the after-effects. One of the
more dramatic was self-induced vomiting, which often allowed
the binge to continue. Binges were usually followed by awe-
some distress and expressions of the most bitter self-condemnation, usually focused on the eating itself, and rarely on
inter-personal concerns. Finally, the binge and the later guilt
were often followed by quixotically austere diets, usually of
very short duration.

Together Mr. Cohen and I began to recognize these
eating binges as discrete events, identifying when they occurred, how long they lasted, and what happened afterward.
Now we turned to the next question. What started them?

It had been relatively easy to discover the characteristics
and consequences of the binges themselves; it was much harder
to find a pattern in what preceded them. But the search was
important. For understanding the events that precipitate eating binges led, often quite directly, to understanding the major
problems in a patient's life. And sometimes the solutions to
these problems led to control of their obesity.

Trying to discover the cause of Mr. Cohen's eating binges
seemed at first quite hopeless. Practically everything he did
appeared to bring on a binge. He would binge whenever he
cashed a check and had money in his hand, or whenever he
went to the Household Finance Corporation and came out
with a loan. He would binge to reward himself after he finished
a hard job. He would binge to celebrate when he had signed

up a new student for tutoring. He would binge when he felt "down in the dumps and didn't give a damn," or when he was feeling expansive, "like a Kwakiutl Indian giving a potlatch."

But gradually, as the binges became less frequent, Mr. Cohen learned to focus his attention more and more sharply upon the period preceding them. Slowly, over a period of many weeks, a pattern began to appear.

In retrospect, there had been clues as early as the third visit. Looking back at my notes for that hour, I saw a remark that had struck me at the time. In describing his over-eating, Mr. Cohen had said, "There is this curious feeling, sometimes, that I'm getting even with someone. It's a vague feeling and it sounds queer to me. I don't know who I'm angry at, or why."

After a pause he had gone on to say that he got angry at his mother when she seemed to disapprove of his eating. "And then I ate as if I meant to spite her."

The second clue came from the binge after his visit to Minsky's burlesque; this was the first time he had referred to problems with his wife. He had made the casual comment that "naturally" he couldn't tell her about the burlesque show. And he went on to talk about his dream years before of nude girls dancing in the subway, and how he associated the dream with marital troubles. Finally, and most importantly, he spoke of his feelings about having been left out of the pornographic picture show because of his prudish remarks which had followed his wife's lead.

As we discussed these events over the next few weeks, it became apparent that not only had Hyman Cohen felt left out, he had felt intense resentment. Most of all he had been distressed at his own passivity in having followed his wife's lead, and in having expressed sentiments about the pornography that were almost the opposite of those he really felt.

We gradually learned that anger played a critical role in his binges; and, as treatment continued, he became more aware of this anger. One incident was particularly instructive.

He had been given the responsibility of disciplining a fourteen year-old boy who had a record of truancy. The boy had defied Mr. Cohen, who suddenly found himself slapping him. "I don't know how it happened. I didn't have the vaguest thought of doing anything like that. But when I saw that little monster sneering at me, I guess I just lost control. I didn't mean to hit him. I just wanted to overawe him. But when he looked so defiant, I just got furious." Then, with a casualness which belied the significance of his remark, he said, "If I hadn't hit that boy, I know I would have gone out and had a binge."

The next week, by contrast, he got angry on two occasions and had not been able to do anything about the anger. He arrived for his appointment three pounds heavier.

By the time Mr. Cohen was able to embark upon a serious, sustained diet, his relationship with his wife had begun to deteriorate. This unfortunate development had one favorable consequence: it greatly facilitated the identification of events that precipitated eating binges. His binges occurred when he had been infuriated by his wife. This fury, however, did not always result in an eating binge. At times it led to physical violence—and twice caused injuries to his wife serious enough to require medical attention. Never after such violence did he have an eating binge.

By the second year of treatment, we could generalize further about the anger which precipitated binges: they usually followed a period during which he had not been able to respond effectively to the person who had angered him. Again and again we recognized situations like that of the party, when his wife had denounced pornography, and when, helpless and passive, he had found himself "selling out" and complying with another's wishes. Later, if he found that these wishes were not in his own best interest, he would feel powerless and betrayed. Mounting anger would set the stage for a binge.

The circumstances that had surrounded his first binges, at the age of 19 or 20, supported the idea that helplessness and passivity in response to threats to his integrity had regu-

larly led to anger and binges. During college he had spent
much of his spare time working in his parents' bakery and
later in a delicatessen. The family had been very poor, and
he had felt humiliated by the poverty and "degraded" by
having to wear an apron in the bakery, "like a shopkeeper,
deferring to the wishes of others."

One event in particular stuck in his mind. When he had
been working in the delicatessen, an Irish Catholic youth had
been dissatisfied with a frankfurter Mr. Cohen had served
him. Voicing his scorn, he threw it at Mr. Cohen, mustard
and all, splattering his clean clothes. "I remember thinking
at the time, 'Here I am, aspiring to a professional career and
having to cater to these crumbs and be subservient to them.
I don't belong here. I am a displaced aristocrat, a member
of the intellectual elite. And yet here I am, having to eat
their shit . . .' "

Instead, he had eaten cakes and cookies. In those days,
when his eating binges had had their start, Mr. Cohen ate
what was at hand. In the delicatessen, a cake, possibly two,
had served as a starter, followed by cookies, crackers, "anything at all," all washed down with a quart of milk.

The detail of Hyman Cohen's eating pattern, and the
larger symptomatic picture into which it fell, formed the basis
of my lecture at the psychiatric hospital. In it I described
the night-eating pattern and contrasted it with the binge-eating pattern so well-exemplified by Hyman Cohen.

Afterwards, over coffee, the informal discussion became
quite animated. "I don't get it," a tall dark young staff member remarked. "A friend of yours, a layman, refers a patient
to you and tells you he is a compulsive eater. You treat him
for two years and you end up with the conclusion that he
is a compulsive eater. What's the big deal?"

Yes, it did appear that Mr. Cohen was a compulsive
eater. But that was not the point I was trying to make. I
was attempting to describe particular kinds of behavior so
discrete and clearly defined that everyone could agree upon
them. And I was hoping to use these descriptions of eating
behavior to classify different kinds of human obesity.

The rather diffuse concept of compulsive eating provided a good example. By contrast, the notion of binge-eating is quite definite. While it is fairly easy to decide whether a person is a binge-eater, it may be very difficult to decide whether he is a compulsive eater. On the simplest level, "compulsion" is a descriptive term. It refers to a strong, often irresistible, inclination to carry out repetitive and often apparently meaningless acts. A well-known example is the hand-washing compulsion that drives people to wash their already clean hands 20, 30 and 40 times a day for no reason that they can recognize.

Some obese people do appear subject to strong inclinations to eat, and even over-eat, and Mr. Cohen was certainly a good example of this. But almost anyone who has gone without food for a time is strongly inclined to eat, and normal-weight people may be even more strongly inclined than many obese ones. When "compulsive eating" is defined in these older, descriptive terms, it accounts for the over-eating of no more than a small minority of obese people.

But compulsions can also be considered in terms of the psychic apparatus which is presumed to underlie them. According to this view, the origins of compulsions are found in the conflict between a drive and the defense mechanisms opposed to that drive. Under appropriate circumstances, the intensity of the conflict is decreased by isolating the psychic energy attached to the drive and displacing it onto some neutral topic. For example, the intensity of a hostile drive towards a husband may be decreased by displacing the energy which activates it onto a neutral act such as hand-washing. The conflict-ridden housewife thereby becomes less tense in the presence of her husband, but at the expense of repetitive, apparently meaningless, hand-washing.

This is the sort of compulsion which seemed to precipitate Mr. Cohen's eating binges, and understanding them appeared helpful in his treatment. But it had taken a great deal of hard work to reach this point. And it seemed unlikely that the diagnosis of compulsive eating could be made in anyone without a similarly arduous effort. If so, we are able to discover who is a compulsive eater only by a process so cumbersome that we will probably never be able to identify more than a few of them.

What are the implications of eating binges? What does this diagnosis tell us about the kind of person who binges and the hope of controlling his obesity? How many obese people are binge-eaters? It is clearly an uncommon disorder, and it is difficult for any one investigator to draw conclusions about it from the limited number of binge-eaters he is likely to encounter. I have carefully studied no more than nine or ten.

In the course of this work, I have been surprised to discover that binge-eating is not confined to obese people. It is even more commonly associated with anorexia nervosa, a rare disorder that afflicts primarily females, particularly adolescents, who voluntarily restrict their food intake so uncompromisingly that many become walking skeletons and some even die. As many as 50 percent may eat in binges. In fact, the frightening experience of losing control and gorging on food seems to play a large part in the rigid restrictions these young women put upon their eating. Some say that they feel that the slightest freedom in eating would result in a total loss of control. And the diets they undertake with such drastic effect are often frighteningly austere, even bizarre, surpassing in intensity those of obese binge-eaters. It is perhaps not surprising that many of them have a morbid fear of becoming obese.

Fortunately, there is a paradox about binge-eating which offers some grounds for optimism regarding treatment. Binge-eaters usually have severe emotional disturbances, which are little helped by the emotional support of family, friends and physicians—or even by extensive weight reduction. Yet the results of treatment (of the few who have undergone prolonged psychotherapy) have been surprisingly good. The treatment has frequently been stormy and always prolonged. But a few binge-eaters have not only resolved their emotional difficulties, they have lost a great deal of weight in the process.

The binges themselves may even be an asset, for an understanding of the events which cause eating binges fre-

quently leads directly to the major conflicts which disturb
the patient.

four
Physical Activity

Hyman Cohen's story did not end with the study of binge-eating, nor was it ever confined to that inquiry. Over the 14 years that he was my patient, many concerns influenced his treatment. An important one was the extent of his physical activity.

The relationship between physical activity and obesity is a fascinating one. There is a large folklore about how inactive—"lazy" is the usual term—obese people are. But it took modern physiological research to demonstrate that it is possible for an animal to become obese as a result solely of its inactivity. Some kinds of hereditarily obese animals actually eat less than littermates whose weight is perfectly normal. Could some obese people similarly become obese simply from inactivity?

Research with such animals suggests how this could occur. If normal weight rats are provided varying amounts of exercise in a running wheel, they regulate their body weight quite precisely, so long as they get at least an hour of exercise per day. For every hour of increased activity they increase the amount of food they eat by an amount just sufficient to compensate for the additional calories that are burned up in work. As a result their body weight remains constant.

When the physical activity of the rats falls below one hour a day, however, the results change in a surprising manner. The less they work, the more they eat! On the other hand, increasing their physical activity (to levels of no more than the critical one hour a day) causes them to eat *less*.

The effects upon body weight are predictable. Decreasing physical activity and increasing food intake leads to a rapid gain in weight. Conversely, rats whose physical activity is increased (to no more than an hour a day), and whose appetites decreased, lose weight.

This is really a remarkable finding. Its unexpected, paradoxical quality, so characteristic of great discoveries, continues to intrigue me. I cannot help but feel that we have still not realized all of its implications. But some of them were clear from the beginning.

We already know that the great increase in obesity in our affluent society has not resulted simply from the greater availability of food. Adequate amounts of food have been available for large segments of our population for many years. The widespread decrease in physical activity seems a more likely cause, as one mechanical device after the other has taken over the tasks formerly carried out by human muscles.

But until research with animals on activity and obesity, it had not been apparent how this decrease in physical activity led to obesity. If people were regulating their body weight correctly, the decrease in physical activity should have been accompanied by an equivalent decrease in the amount they ate. Evidently this wasn't happening. But why not?

We can assume that the answer lies in our technological advances. In the United States of many years ago, as in many underdeveloped areas today, the activity level of most people was probably high enough to cause a more or less automatic regulation of their food intake (like the rats who ran more than one hour a day). With greater technological development, however, our physical activity may have fallen to whatever is the human equivalent of the rats' running less than one hour a day. And like the sedentary rats, our decreased physical activity may actually be increasing our eating.

If these assumptions are even approximately correct, they are bright with promise for the control of obesity. They suggest that an increase in physical activity may help to control obesity, not just because of the extra calories burned up, but more importantly, by moving obese people back to the level where food intake is more instinctively related to physical activity.

As striking as these findings were, it was well over a year after learning of them before I started to work on the topic. Much as I had wanted to earlier, I had no idea of where to begin. Then one day on impulse I dropped into an instrument store whose window display had long intrigued me. I had always wanted an excuse to buy one of the shiny, fascinating and overpriced instruments which were so artfully displayed. Behind a pocket-watch sized instrument was the sign: "Pedometer. Find out how far you walk. Wear it on the golf course or at work. Amaze your family and friends." Without a moment's hesitation I bought one; and since that first purchase, I have regularly used pedometers, measuring my own activity daily for 3 years, and my patients' for even longer.

In the initial study of physical activity, we used a sentence-completion test. It consisted of 15 paired, open-ended sentence fragments, half of which used the first person pronoun and half of which used the third person pronoun.

From the first we suspected that depression might play a part in attitudes towards activity, and we prepared the beginning of sentences to test this idea. "When I am blue, I . . ." explored the subjects' conscious appraisal of what they would do when depressed. The same inquiry was worded in the third person: "When she's down in the dumps, she . . ." We had

found that, through this third-person device we could sometimes uncover attitudes which subjects would be too self-
conscious to admit in the first person.

We confined the study to obese women, who outnum-
bered men by 9 to 1 in the hospital clinics. We reviewed the
records of these patients to exclude any who had some physical
disability other than obesity, which might affect their physical
activity. We were surprised at how few there were. The
overwhelming proportion of obese people who sought medical
attention had no associated physical disabilities.

When we compared the activity of those obese women
with that of a control group of matched, non-obese women,
we found a striking difference. The obese women were far
less active than the non-obese women. Whereas the latter
walked 4.5 miles a day, the obese women walked no more
than 1.5.

The sentence-completion test showed differences which
were almost as marked. Sentences probing the women's response to depression were particularly impressive. Every one
of the obese women reported a passive acceptance of a depressed mood. Typical responses were: "When I am blue, I
just cry," and "When she is down in the dumps, she *just sulks.*"
The non-obese women, on the other hand, frequently gave
responses which indicated that they were struggling against
feelings of despondency. Typical ones were: "When I am blue,
I *clean house,*" and "When she is down in the dumps, she *counts
her blessings.*"

We had also attempted to assess the subjects' attitudes
toward boredom, a complaint which I had heard all too often
from obese patients. Again the results indicated more passive
responses on the part of the obese women: "When I am not
interested, I *get depressed,*" and "When she's bored, she *often
shows it.*" Although some of the non-obese women gave similar
responses, the majority replied in a more active vein: "When
I am not interested, I *read,*" and "When she's bored, she *irons
clothes.*"

Social interaction is a major stimulus to physical activity,
and we therefore tried to assess the subjects' attitudes toward

it. Again we found significant differences between the two groups. The obese women usually gave responses suggesting far less capacity to develop easy relationships with other people: "Working with people makes me feel *no different than working alone,"* and "The others in the office make her feel *isolated."* The non-obese women, on the other hand, evidenced a remarkable degree of confidence in their ability to form good social relations. Typical responses were: "Working with people makes me feel *just perfect,"* and "The others in the office make her feel *welcome."*

These clear-cut results elated us. This was the first study to actually measure the physical activity of obese people, and it showed clearly the part played by lessened physical activity. Furthermore, the correlation between activity and attitudes suggested that any attempt to increase physical activity was going to have to deal with the self-defeating attitudes of the obese. Prominent among these attitudes were those indicating depression. Did depression lie behind the inactivity of obese people? One way of approaching the problem was to measure their levels of physical activity over a period of time and see if these related to the presence and intensity of their depression.

Once again I turned to my patients. Would they be willing to wear a pedometer and keep a record of their physical activity? Everyone whom I asked agreed, and I immediately began to keep daily records of their physical activity.

This was where Hyman Cohen proved particularly helpful. From our second meeting on, he had repeatedly asked if he could take part in some kind of research. For a time I had demurred, trying to understand his reasons. But I finally decided that his self-esteem would be buoyed by viewing himself as a collaborator in medical research. And I was coming to the conclusion that his treatment was going to be a long one, allowing plenty of time to work out any complications engendered by the dual relationship.

During the first weeks of treatment, Mr. Cohen walked no more than 2.0 miles a day. As he explained it, "You have no idea how lazy I am, Doc. I've got a card catalogue in

my office and when I'm working on it lots of times I'll send
for a student messenger to get the cards rather than walk
across the room . . . Why I'll take the car if I've only got
three blocks to go, even if I have to park so far away from
where I am going that I'll have to walk more than three
blocks to get there. I'm that lazy."

We spent a good deal of time talking about his inactivity,
and he attributed much of it to his sweating. "You see, I
sweat so easily, Doc, especially when I exercise, and all that
sweat just makes me feel uncomfortable. It chafes my skin
too, especially around the crotch, and I would do anything
rather than sweat."

Very soon after Mr. Cohen began to keep a record of
his physical activity, there occurred the significant events
surrounding his trip to the burlesque show and the explosive
eating binge which had followed. The pedometer measurements during this brief period told a striking story: During
the nine days before the fateful party at which he supported
his wife's condemnation of pornography, Mr. Cohen had
walked an average of 2.1 miles a day. For the following three
days he kept no record of his activity. Then followed six days
of depression with an average of 0.5 mile a day. On the day
of the eating binge his activity returned to its former level;
and during the next nine days, with the lifting of the depression, he again walked an average of 2.1 miles a day.

Here was a very close association between a severely
depressed mood (superimposed on a more chronic depression)
and a marked reduction in physical activity. Not being invited
to watch the pornographic movies had been a devastating
blow on three counts. First, Mr. Cohen was a sexually very
active man with a strong fascination for all aspects of the
topic. He would have liked nothing better than to watch the
pornographic movies. Second, he had at least the usual sensitivity to rejection, and he felt doubly rejected because the
friends who had invited him to a conventional party had
excluded him from a gathering in which he would have had
a far greater interest. Third, and most important, was his
betrayal of himself. He was well aware of his intense curiosity

about sex. His prudish protestations, in imitation of his wife's, had been a shameless sell-out.

It was only later in treatment that I began to understand this passivity toward his wife and his inability to acknowledge what seemed to be strong evidence of hostility toward her. Some further description of Hyman Cohen and his past may help explain the reasons.

Hyman Cohen was the older of two sons born in New York to a Jewish immigrant couple from Eastern Europe. He maintained that he had no memories before the age of eight, and at no time during our long association did I find any evidence to contradict this unusual assertion. So I was unable to ascertain early childhood influences upon his later behavior. But even earlier influences, genetic ones, seemed to play a role.

His father was very obese and suffered from a manic depressive psychosis which hospitalized him for the last 30 years of his life. His mother was also obese, and the obesity of the two made it unlikely that he would escape the condition. He did escape the mental deterioration which afflicted his father and was never hospitalized. But throughout his life he showed milder manic depressive features: a strong tendency to elation or, less frequently, depression; the ability to deny undeniable problems; and a lack of sensitivity (or psychological-mindedness).

Mr. Cohen's earliest memory was when his father had left home. He remembered his mother telling him about it and recalled his mixed feelings—sadness at his father's leaving, but pride at what his mother told him his father was going to do. She apparently had controlled her disappointment and told her baseball-loving son that his father had moved west to manage the Detroit Tigers. He learned much later that his father had been fired from his job after a fight with his boss, and had left town to work as a traveling salesman.

The other memories were bitter ones. There was the time when his father could not answer a neighbor who asked what grade his son was in. On another occasion, when he had declined his father's invitation to go to a boxing match, his father ferociously scolded him "for not being a red-blooded American boy."

But the bitterest disappointment occurred when he was 17 years old. Hyman Cohen had undergone an appendectomy and was waiting in the hospital, when he was surprised by the appearance of his father, who he had thought was out of town. His father bundled him into the car to drive him home, and when they arrived, let him out of the car, and drove on to park it. When Mr. Cohen went to the front door, he found himself too weak to open it, and he waited for his father to return and open it for him. But his father never came, and he finally sat down in front of the house and cried. "I felt helpless and completely neglected by my father. It was just the worst time in my life. And that's what started my weight problem. I just decided that I would eat and eat until I had built my strength up. And of course I just didn't stop."

Actually Mr. Cohen had been overweight most of his life, but it became more severe after this incident; and it was this incident which he came to view as a specific cause of his obesity.

"After that, Dad appeared only very briefly, and not very often. I remember he once appeared in a tremendous old green Lincoln touring car with a Negro chauffeur. He was walking around the neighborhood telling people about the big business deals he was making and borrowing money from them. This was very embarrassing to my mother and me, and the store wasn't doing very well either."

Mr. Cohen was 19 the last time his father appeared. "Sometimes he would be very dapper and well-dressed. But this time he wasn't. He looked terrible. He was dirty and had a beard, and a dead cigar butt in his mouth that he kept chewing on. He wasn't making much sense, and then he tried to assault Mother sexually. I had to threaten him with a baseball bat to get him to let her alone. We had to commit him then, and I don't think this was the first time. But he never got out of the hospital after that."

Mr. Cohen's memories of his mother were less unreservedly negative. They weren't really joyful memories either—I sometimes thought of them as bitter-sweet. "I guess the happiest memories of my life were of times with Mother. I must have been about 13, I can't remember exactly, and my mother had a job in a candy store out in Throgg's Neck. The high point of my week was going out there by trolley on Saturday night and helping her put together the Sunday papers and then coming back with her on the trolley after midnight on Sunday."

Mr. Cohen often told me about these Saturday nights, and he kept coming back to them. "I can fix one date around that time very accurately, the closing of the banks in March of 1933. I have a clear recollection of my parents standing in line for many hours trying to withdraw their account."

Throughout Mr. Cohen's youth financial difficulties plagued the family, and his mother never escaped from the frightened, penurious world of those days. She was always worrying about money. Many years later when Mr. Cohen bought his first car, his mother was terribly upset and begged him again and again to be more careful with his money.

After one of the occasions when his father lost his job, there was a large family meeting to plot the proper course for his parents. It was decided that they should run a bakery, and his mother's family bought it for them. "That was a confused and uncomfortable period. It must have been about that time that Dad left home and had some sort of a job as a traveling salesman. We moved in with some of my mother's family in very crowded conditions up in the Bronx.

"Then I can remember another family conference. It was very tense. My uncle Sam threatened to beat Dad up if he didn't do better. I remember he said he'd beat the be-Jesus out of him. Then they loaned my mother $1700 to buy the bakery. We kept living with her sisters and her mother all of this time, and it was terribly hard work. We'd open up at six in the morning and stay open till midnight. There wasn't any family life at all. And that went on for seven years."

Mr. Cohen's account of a childhood lived in close relationship to food stores is a very common one among obese men. It has seemed to me that a majority of them have either

been raised by a family involved with a food business, or
have had a food-related occupation themselves, or both. Of
course this was not so unusual in New York, from which most
of my patients originally came, and where there is such a
profusion of small confectionary shops. These are often run
by Jews, and obesity in Jewish men and boys is not unusual.
For women the association between food occupations and
obesity is not nearly so close. One can speculate that this
is because the average woman has so much more to do with
food in the course of her personal daily routine.

Despite all the turmoil of these years, Mr. Cohen gradu-
ated from high school and started college. But financial pressures soon forced him to cut down to one course at college
in order to help his mother with the bakery. He was pursuing
this dual career at the age of 19 when his father had returned
home for the last time. Perhaps his father's hospitalization
ended any hope of improvement in the family finances. In
any event, his mother sold the bakery to pay for her son to
attend college full time. She got a job working in a sister's
delicatessen (and was still working there during the time I
treated her son).

Such devotion on the part of his mother might have
repaired Mr. Cohen's loss of his father. But the days with
Mother were not all bliss—and not simply because of her
financial insecurities. When Mr. Cohen was 8 years old, the
year that his father had first left home, his mother had had
a second son. And this son received most of what his mother
liked to call her "love." From Hyman she had demanded
companionship and performance; he had been flattered, and
had complied. From his brother she demanded nothing except
the chance to give. Or, as Hyman Cohen's wife was later
to remark in her acid manner, "If you were her husband,
your brother was her lover."

Mr. Cohen grew up with an intense jealousy of this
spoiled young darling and a lifelong impairment of his ability
to relate to younger men and boys. His experience with his
father had left him with a hopeless yearning and a real despair
of ever being able to trust an older man. Clearly, these emo-

tions underlay his identification with his psychiatrist and his intense dependence upon him.

But basically Mr. Cohen looked to women for his security, and his search was desperate, unrelenting and compulsive. Despite his puritanical background and its financial strictures, he had begun to make the rounds of prostitutes long before he had emerged from adolescence. And graduation from college and entry into wartime military service had signaled the onset of almost frantic sexual activity. Until the age of 23 all of this activity was with prostitutes.

Then, one day when he was on furlough, forlorn and homesick, he met a "nice girl" and she took him to bed. "I married her three weeks later, out of gratitude. What else could I do?" In response to my raised eyebrows, he continued, "It was the first time I had ever had sex without having to pay for it. I just felt so grateful to her that I didn't know what to do. The least I could do was marry her."

Mr. Cohen's attitude toward his wife had this intense, all-or-nothing quality. His relationship with her was for many years one of unqualified awe. The first time he ever mentioned her to me he said, "When I diet she praises me, and that makes me feel like a good boy."

The bliss of the marriage cooled when his wife proposed that they have a child, and things went downhill as the proposal became a demand. For five years he put her off, and her demands mounted. Finally, when Mr. Cohen was 28 years old, his wife played her trump card. Unless they had a child, she would leave him.

"It was just awful. I couldn't live without her and yet I couldn't stand the idea of being a father, I just wasn't ready to be a father, and she forced me into it." For a time after the birth of their son, Mr. Cohen had left his wife, but he had crept back to her within a few weeks, contrite and unhappy.

Over the years they had settled into an equilibrium of unhappy mutual dependency. Only as we began to examine the marriage in the course of treatment did he realize just how unhappy they were.

The marriage never really survived the birth of their son, Walter. Mr. Cohen was never able to shake the deep conviction that his wife preferred Walter to him, and would have left him had it not been for his siring her child. He felt insecure, apprehensive, depressed. He felt betrayed at having to be a father, and constantly avoided his son. And he treated his wife as the betrayer, at times passively complaining to her, at others actively shouting and even hitting her—all the while ridiculing her increasingly neurotic behavior. His wife, in turn, found that a child did not bring relief from her intense suffering. Now she had to cope with her baby alone, with no help from her increasingly estranged husband. Adventurous and highly intelligent as a young woman, she found herself restricted to a narrow round of household chores, which she carried out with mounting desperation.

It had struck me during Mr. Cohen's first mention of his wife, when he was describing their happy marriage, that he had laughed as he told me about how he frequently tried to choke her during his sleep. He similarly told me cheerful accounts of her "little rituals." One was to say "God keep Hyman safe," ten times before going to sleep—five times if they had had intercourse—and of her panic if he prevented enactment of the ritual.

It seemed as though that was the first time he had ever thought about the meaning of his wife's waxing the floors every day and her refusal to permit either shoes or bare feet on them; only slippers would protect the shiny luster of the floors she polished so religiously, and she would go into fits of screaming if her son walked on them in his bare feet. Mr. Cohen had long since given up hope of any such freedom.

He had never related the events in his daily life to the fluctuations in his weight, and it was difficult to reconstruct the relationships at this late date. After the experience of his father's abandonment following his appendectomy at age 17, Mr. Cohen's eating had soon brought his weight to 220 pounds. And there it remained through the military service which followed college. After he was released, at the age of

25, it had risen to nearly the 272 pounds which he weighed when he came to see me at the age of 37. This increase had been punctuated by frequent diets. And it was apparently the failure of one of these, and the consequent rapid increase in weight, which had caused him to seek treatment. He was depressed, over-eating and under-active—averaging only two miles a day.

By the time Hyman Cohen had finished telling me about his life, it was easy to understand his compliance with his wife's distaste for the pornographic movies, and his inability to acknowledge his strong hostility toward her. He was so terribly dependent upon her, and so uncertain of her support, that he did not dare to acknowledge even the slightest resentment. He could not be even appropriately self-assertive, for fear that such action might jeopardize that relationship. Locked in their unhappy embrace, the Cohens moved slowly towards tragedy.

The impact of treatment became apparent quite early. First there was a lessening in the intensity of Mr. Cohen's depression. There were also glimmerings of a reduced dependence upon his wife, and the first hints of criticism of her. The following months saw continuing improvement in his mood and a growing independence of his wife. His physical activity, however, increased only slightly, from 2 to 2.5 miles a day, and his weight remained at 270 pounds.

What led to this improvement? I attributed much of it to the strong positive transference which Mr. Cohen had developed towards me. It appeared that his dependent needs were being gratified, and he strongly identified with me, viewing us as fellow explorers in the trackless waste of obesity. I am inclined to believe that this kind of improvement will usually occur in the course of psychotherapy, provided the therapist does not interfere with it.

It was about this time, five months into Hyman Cohen's treatment, that I was offered an excellent position in the Department of Psychiatry at the University of Pennsylvania. Since the job promised new and exciting possibilities, I accepted, and made plans to leave New York.

The move to Pennsylvania brought with it one of the most painful moments in a physician's life—parting from his patients. For some, termination of treatment was possible. For others, transfer to the care of another doctor seemed the wisest course. Hyman Cohen was among this second group. And one spring morning, I told him that I had discussed the situation with an excellent psychiatrist in New York, who would be happy to see him for treatment. I had developed a real affection for Hyman Cohen, and I told him how sorry I was that this development would end our relationship, one I had come to prize. Although I did not say it, I felt particularly unhappy at demonstrating to him once again the unreliability of older men, always leaving him when they were needed most.

Mr. Cohen's reaction to my departure was, in retrospect, understandable. He swallowed his disappointment and told me that if we only had two months left, he intended to make the most of it. He had no desire at all to see another doctor, and "I have decided here and now that I will get down to work and finish up this treatment in the two months that we have left."

It almost looked as if he were going to do just that. He came into the office the next week beaming, to announce that the preceding week had been the most successful since the start of treatment—in fact, one of the most successful he had ever known. He had embarked upon a reducing diet and had already lost six pounds, and he had begun to make a conscious effort to increase his physical activity.

These feelings of well-being continued and grew into what he called his "benzedrine syndrome." His energy became boundless, his need for sleep dropped to less than five hours a day, and everything took on a rosy glow. "It's like magic—your prediction has come true. Just by understanding my reactions, I can control my eating with no difficulty at all. It just isn't a struggle any more. Things which would have thrown me now slide off my back with no trouble. Even my wife says that now she believes in psychiatry. It really works. She has mentioned my nails growing out for the first time since she's known me, and how I can control my appetite, and she says that this is the best that she can remember."

He continued to diet, dropping from 270 to 250 pounds in six weeks. His activity shot up from 2.5 to 4.5 miles a day, an astonishing increase for him. He was clearly reacting to the threatened loss with his usual pattern of elation, and for a time I was worried about him. The circumstances seemed too similar to the first elated stage of a dieting depression.

Then Mr. Cohen took matters into his own hands. On our next-to-last appointment he began somewhat hesitantly by saying that he had had a talk about my impending departure with the friend who referred him to me. Mr. Liebowitz had suggested that he ask if he could come down to Philadelphia to see me. "So I'm putting the question to you, Doc." I told him that I would be glad to see him in Philadelphia, but pointed out some of the difficulties. He replied that since school was already finished for the year there would be no difficulty in his getting away from New York. We agreed to try it out for the summer and then see how feasible it was to continue after that.

This direct action towards a course which he desired, and its favorable outcome, had a strong impact upon Mr. Cohen. His self-confidence soared, and with it came an end to the elation. His mood fell to a more appropriate level; he began to sleep more regularly and for longer periods; and his hyper-activity decreased. Pedometer measurements fell from 4.5 miles a day to 3 miles a day, and they stayed at this level for as long as he continued to make these measurements, a period of over two years. His weight also leveled off at 250 pounds and continued at this level for several years.

In reviewing these long-term records of physical activity and weight, I felt that they supported the findings of the research on physical activity and obesity in rats, which I described above. Early in treatment, when he was averaging 2 miles a day, Mr. Cohen's weight had fluctuated around 270 pounds. Six months later, when his physical activity had stabilized at 3 miles a day, his weight also stabilized, at 250 pounds. Neither of these measures showed appreciable long-term changes during the tumultuous period which followed.

This period was ushered in, paradoxically, by Mr. Cohen's steady progress in treatment. For this progress seemed to disturb his wife, who became increasingly distraught and apprehensive. The precarious equilibrium between them eroded. As his increasing capacity for independence freed him from his dependence on her, she became more and more disturbed. A year of alcoholism was followed by another year of increasingly bizarre behavior and periodic psychiatric hospitalizations. Three years after her husband had entered treatment, Mrs. Cohen committed suicide.

Mr. Cohen continued treatment with me over a period of 14 years, at first on a weekly basis, and later at infrequent intervals. And occasional letters keep me in touch with him to this day.

The years of turmoil were followed by years of loneliness. Gradually, however, Mr. Cohen came to accept his son and even to love him. Then he married a warm and loving woman and began the relationship which Mr. Cohen still feels is the best thing that ever happened to him. He qualified for the job as principal of his high school and for many years has coped well with the rigorous demands of this office. Throughout these years his weight has remained around 250 pounds.

The treatment of Hyman Cohen, which swept me into the tragedy and triumphs of his life, moved me deeply. It left me with a growing dissatisfaction with a therapy which could help an individual only at such a high cost to his family. And it raised serious doubts about the importance of mood-related changes in physical activity.

On the one hand, it was clear that depression was associated with decreases in physical activity. This combination had occurred so frequently and under so many different circumstances, that I no longer doubted that the two factors were linked. On the other hand, the comparative size of the changes in activity during depression was disappointingly small. Mr. Cohen walked 2 miles a day when he was depressed and 3 miles a day when he was not depressed. This 50 percent increase was highly significant from a statistical point of view; but in practical terms of increased calorie expenditure, it was far less impressive. It was only an extra twenty minutes of walking, no more than 200 Calories.

Some of the short-term periods of depression—such as the one which followed the disappointment about the pornographic movies—were associated with an even more severe reduction in physical activity. And the combination of depression and diminished physical activity probably made some contribution to his obesity. But the contrast between this contribution and others made it clear that other influences were far more important. The years of study and the collection of thousands of pedometer measurements provided a number of hunches as to what some of these influences were, and sufficient data to test them.

There seemed to be three sets of influences on physical activity: the emotional, which I had explored with disappointing results, the biological, and the social. Among the biological influences, there was the intriguing possibility that environmental temperature exerted an impact, for it had been shown to have marked effects upon the physical activity of experimental animals: lowering temperature increases physical activity, and raising it reduces activity. And obese people are unusually susceptible to the discomforts of heat and humidity. Anyone who has spent much time with obese people knows how miserable they feel during hot weather, and how even the slightest increase in body heat produced by a meal will often cause profuse sweating. For them a warm spell becomes a heat wave, when minimal physical activity produces the sweating of vigorous exercise.

Spurred by these considerations, we carried out a study which examined, among other things, the relationship of temperature to physical activity. We conducted the study at a nearby Girl Scout camp, supplying both obese and non-obese girls with pedometers: and we recorded their activity levels as heat and humidity rose and fell through the Philadelphia summer. It seemed that we could hardly fail to come up with some positive findings. In fact, I can't remember another study of which I had higher expectations.

But the results were completely negative. Neither heat, nor humidity, nor the temperature-humidity index had the slightest influence upon the physical activity of the girls. It was cold comfort to have a clear-cut negative result, but the study did help to limit our approach: we didn't need to worry about heat and humidity as causes of obesity, at least among young girls.

The next attempt to look at a biological influence on physical activity had a happier outcome, although not in the way I expected. We knew that phases of the reproductive cycle have a potent influence upon the physical activity of female rats. They will run three and even four times as far in a day during one phase of the cycle as they will in another. An influence which could be so powerful in one species must surely have some effect in another.

For a period of nearly two years I tried to show such an effect. More than 30 wives of medical students gamely strapped pedometers to their waists and recorded their activity through three or four menstrual cycles. Their activity did fluctuate wildly from day to day, but never in relation to their menstrual cycle. They did, however, show striking peaks and valleys which corresponded to another cycle—weekdays and weekends. The search for biological influences on physical activity had failed, only to lead to the identification of far more powerful ones: social factors. The largest differences in physical activity which I was to find were those between weekdays and weekends. But the differences were not always in the same direction.

Some active persons with confining jobs showed low weekday activity and a great increase in activity over the weekends, when they could give expression to their natural inclinations. Others, with little natural inclination toward physical activity, might show high levels of activity during the week, when their jobs forced them out of their sedentary ways, with a decrease on weekends. Obese people were far more likely to fall into this second category. Hyman Cohen was a shining example.

Only very rarely did Hyman Cohen walk as far on

a weekend day as he did on a weekday. In fact, during the
first three months of his treatment, he never did. And later,
when his physical activity had stabilized at a rate of 3 miles
a day, he averaged 4 miles a day on weekdays at work and
no more than a mile a day on the weekends. The influence
of the day of the week produced not just large differences
in physical activity, but differences of an order of magnitude
far beyond those produced by emotional factors. Hyman
Cohen's physical activity on weekdays was four times as great
as on weekends. By contrast, the increase in physical activity
associated with recovery from his depression was only 50 percent.

I meditated on these figures long and hard. The story
they told was as straightforward as any I had found since
I had started studying obesity. It was not a story that was
congenial to the notions I had started with. For as I reluctantly
began to realize, these figures made one thing clear: a simple
social fact had a far stronger influence on physical activity
than anything that I ever had found in the study of stress
and disease.

What were other social factors that might influence physical activity? Clearly occupation was one. Our study of obese
women had shown that most who gave their occupations as
"housewife" were remarkably inactive. But, since most of our
subjects were housewives, it was impossible to assess the influence of occupation on physical activity. It occurred to me
that among men, on the other hand, the very wide spread
of occupations should make it possible to do a careful quanti-
tative study on the influence of occupation upon physical
activity. So we set about the study of obesity in men.

Our very first interviews with obese men provided an
interesting confirmation of the importance of physical activity
in the regulation of body weight. Eight of our first sample of
men had served in the Army and had undergone the less than
rigorous basic training of the peacetime Army. Nevertheless,
they had lost an average of 20 pounds. No one lost less than ten
pounds; and some lost as much as 30. Furthermore, each of
these men had gained weight following basic training, and

almost all had returned to their previous obese states within a
few months of assignment to sedentary garrison life.

We were particularly interested in the reasons which
these men gave for their weight losses and weight gains. Everyone attributed the weight loss to the increase in physical
activity. None reported any conscious effort at restricting the
amount he ate nor any shortage of food. All said that they
had lost weight with no effort at all, eating just as much
as they wished.

The accounts of these men made it clear that there was a
significant increase in their caloric output during basic training. Was this increased output sufficient to account for their
weight loss? Or did the increased physical activity result in an
actual decrease in the amount they ate? And conversely, had
the weight gain following basic training been due solely to a
decrease in physical activity, or had there been an increase in
eating?

None of the men could remember enough of the details
of the food they ate to allow us to reconstruct their caloric
intake. But they reported, with remarkable unanimity, that
the weight loss during basic training had occurred with none
of the discomfort of their other weight-loss experiences. All
remembered quite well that they had lost weight despite the
freedom to eat as much as they wanted. So we had clear
evidence that increases in activity had not been matched by
commensurate increases in eating, despite complete freedom
to eat as much as desired.

It has often seemed to me that the simple observations
of this group of men, obtained at so little cost, may contain
more information and provide more guidance for weight reduction than other studies I have carried out at far greater
expense.

After these interviews we easily and quickly carried out
pedometer measurements of the physical activity of 25 obese
and non-obese men. The obese men surprised us by the extent
of their physical activity. On the average they walked over
twice as far as the obese women—4.0 miles compared to 1.5
miles for the obese women. Furthermore, they were very nearly

as active as the non-obese men, who walked no more than 4.5 miles a day. When allowance was made for the greater number of calories burned by the obese as a result of their greater body weight, it became clear that they expended just as many calories as the non-obese men.

This study thus produced another solid finding: gender made a difference. The decreased physical activity and passive attitudes towards it, which had so clearly characterized obese women, were not found in obese men.

These differences in physical activity between obese men and women raised the question as to whether the inactivity of the women was a function of their gender or of the social influences affecting women. In other words, are obese women inactive solely because they are female or because they play a woman's role in society?

To answer this question we had carried out the study mentioned before, at the Girl Scout camp. We had measured the activity and the body weights of the girls at camp, and then again after their return to their more sedentary home life. Consequently we had the data to assess the same group in situations calling for vastly different amounts of physical activity.

Our first question was whether the obese girls were less active than the non-obese girls; were they more like adult women or more like adult men in this respect? The results showed them to be more like the men. At home the obese girls walked 3.5 miles a day; the non-obese walked 5.0 miles a day. When allowance was made for the differing rates of caloric expenditure, the obese girls actually expended more energy at home than did the non-obese girls.

At camp all of the girls had been much more active, and the difference between the groups disappeared. The obese girls walked 7.0 miles a day, the non-obese 7.3 miles a day. The caloric expenditure of the obese girls as a result of physical activity was thus considerably higher than that of the non-obese girls.

Here was a fascinating surprise. In sharp contrast to the obese women we had studied, physical activity played no part in the obesity of these girls. How was this finding to be understood? Did it mean that the activity of obese females decreases as they pass from adolescence into womanhood? Or was our sample of obese girls a biased one, an unusual group which, unlike other obese girls, sought out the active physical and social life of the Girl Scouts? The latter alternative seemed the more plausible. But there was no way of knowing. And we turned our attention to the critical question—did a change in physical activity affect body weight? Did summer camp have the same effect as basic training?

The answer was yes! The obese girls lost weight when compared to the non-obese girls. How did this come about?

For an answer to this question we turned to ratings of appetite recorded by the girls themselves. The difference between obese and non-obese girls was striking. Most of the non-obese girls reported an increase in appetite at camp, probably in response to the increased physical activity. On the other hand, few of the obese girls reported any increase in appetite, and some even reported a decrease. Presumably the actual food intakes, which we were not able to measure, showed the same pattern.

Taken together, the findings of physical activity, appetite, and weight change provide strong support for the theory from the studies with rats. Among the somewhat more active non-obese girls, the move to active camp life had resulted in increased appetite, presumably greater food intake, and little change in body weight. Among the more sedentary obese girls, however, the increased physical activity at camp resulted in little or no increase in appetite, presumably little change in food intake, and weight loss.

What lessons had we learned from these studies? Most important was the evidence that physical activity plays a part in the regulation of body weight, and not only by means of the caloric expenditure which it entails. It may play a larger part by decreasing, or at least preventing an increase in food intake, when obese people increase their physical activity.

And the level of physical activity is controlled by social factors to a far greater degree than by biological or emotional factors. Army recruits were more active and lost weight under the influence of the social pressures of basic training; the same phenomena held true for girls under the social pressure of summer camp.

Here at last were the first glimmerings of a successful treatment for obesity. At the least they seemed more fruitful than the old preoccupation with the personal stresses of the obese. And I came increasingly to feel that social influences, more than emotional and biological, are what cause and sustain obesity.

five
Social Class and Obesity

The work with physical activity profoundly changed my outlook. It made me aware for the first time of the vital role of social factors in the production of obesity. But another line of investigation was to change my outlook even more decisively. This research focused directly on the relationship of social class and obesity. It led me still further from theories of stress and disease, with their emphasis on the life history and experience of the individual, and more deeply into the significance of broad community-wide social factors.

The inquiry began with a question which came to preoccupy me increasingly over the years: Are obese people more neurotic than non-obese people? By this time I was in no

doubt as to the extent of neurotic suffering among obese
people. There was a very great amount. I had treated enough
to know how disturbed they could be, and how even obese
people who seemed on first acquaintance to have few problems, could, when they felt more confident, tell hair-raising
tales of their difficulties. My question was more specific: Did
obese people have more problems than non-obese people?

The route to answering this question was a circuitous one.
It began in a curious way. The Army wanted help in the
treatment of obesity.

The problem had apparently started some time before
when a general had received orders to prepare to move his
division to Germany. This general had commanded troops
there during World War II, and had gained a reputation for
combat effectiveness and for the emphasis he placed on physical fitness. One evening in Washington he was discussing his
forthcoming move overseas with an old friend, who was then
a member of the Joint Chiefs of Staff. While they were reminiscing about their wartime experiences, the division commander confessed how embarrassed he felt about returning
to Germany with his current troops, so far less professional
and less fit than those he had led in combat. The two old
comrades spent some time deploring the deterioration of the
peacetime Army and its lack of physical fitness. When they
came to the subject of fat soldiers they reached unanimity—
neither could stand fat soldiers.

The senior general had asked why the division commander tolerated them, and the latter had protested that he
didn't see that he had a choice. The senior general reportedly
suggested, "Why don't you *order* your fat soldiers to lose
weight? And if they don't obey the order, court martial them."

The division commander said that he would like nothing
better but that he didn't know if he could. The senior general
apparently assured him that he could, and that he would
personally do everything he could to prevent his old buddy
from having to undergo the humiliation of taking fat soldiers
to Germany.

Upon his return to his post the division commander

apparently issued an order that all fat soldiers were to start losing weight at once. Presumably some did; and some did not. After waiting a decent interval, the division commander proceeded to court martial those who did not, on the charge of disobeying an order.

The review of the courts martial was prompt and decisive, and not favorable to the general. He was now to be subjected to the double humiliation of taking fat soldiers to Germany and having his courts martial of these same fat soldiers reversed. He called his old buddy on the Joint Chiefs of Staff, who, in turn, called the Judge Advocate General. The latter explained to the former that obesity was a medical, not a legal problem, and therefore could not be handled by means of court martial. If the senior general wanted something done about it, medical, not legal channels were the appropriate route.

This route was speedily traversed. The senior general called in the Surgeon General and asked him what he intended to do about fat soldiers. The Surgeon General, in turn, called in his staff and relayed the request. Uncertain of how to proceed, but aware that treatment for obesity was unsatisfactory, they approached the Director of Research of the Army Medical Corps for any information about new methods of treatment. Remembering that the Army was contributing a small amount of money for the study of obesity to a program in our clinic, the Director of Research called me.

It was never very clear what the Army wanted. I was assured that they were simply interested in a manual for the treatment of obesity in the Army. I pointed out that it would be difficult to construct a manual without knowing more about the circumstances surrounding the obesity problem. With this in mind, I went to Washington to discuss my contract with its sponsors in the Army Medical Corps.

It was a curious meeting. The two middle-aged captains with whom I spoke acted as if their job were simply to make sure that the technical requirements were met and the amenities observed. As to the fruits of the research, they could not have cared less. And the possibility of conducting a study with Army personnel horrified them.

"That would be quite out of the question, Dr. Stunkard."

"Why?" I asked.

The tall captain began. "Well, you don't understand our situation, what the Army's like today. It's not like it used to be. We've got to be terribly careful. We can't do anything that might offend the men. You can hardly do any kind of studies in the field any more. The first thing you know, some kid gets his nose out of joint and writes his mother, and she gets in touch with her congressman, and we have an investigation on our hands."

Anxious to protect the contract with the Army, and assuming that it was not being given as a form of charity, I tried to think of some study which would warrant continuing support. "What," I asked, "would you think of a study of obesity in men?" A good number of the obese men in any sample would be likely to have had military experience. It might well be possible to learn something about their body weight changes in relation to various aspects of military service. I quickly outlined a research project.

"That sounds like a fine idea," they replied with obvious relief; "just don't get the Army involved." They were beaming as they rose and escorted me to the door. "Thank you for coming to see us, doctor. Just remember, don't get us involved."

Thus was born the research project on "Obesity in Men." The following year, midway through the study, I received a polite letter from the Army which, in one paragraph, thanked me for past services and terminated the contract. By this time I had become so involved in the study that I carried it out anyway.

It involved intensive work with 25 obese men, and a matched number of non-obese men who served as control subjects. We looked for distinctive personality patterns among the obese men and again returned to the question which had begun to obsess me: Are the obese more neurotic than the non-obese?

In short order we were flooded with data; and nowhere

was this embarrassment of riches more embarrassing than in the analysis of the psychological testing. For until that time there had been no standard way of comparing groups on the several dimensions of psychological functioning which were assessed by these tests. As luck would have it, just at that time there appeared a book, *The Interpersonal Diagnosis of Personality,* which provided a general framework for analyzing our psychological test data. Its author was Timothy Leary.

When our study was well underway, I wrote to Dr. Leary and received an invitation to visit him. We spent a pleasant morning discussing the research which each of us was carrying out. As I have since read about Timothy Leary's later life, I have often thought back to that morning and the shy, kindly man who went out of his way to be of help. He seemed pleased that we were using his system in research on obese people, and I was surprised by the deference shown me by this man, already well-established in his field and the author of one of its significant texts.

Dr. Leary described in some detail his goal of collecting a data bank containing detailed psychological tests of groups of similarly afflicted people. As I remember it, he had already collected tests on large numbers of people suffering from asthma and other psychosomatic diseases, as well as on delinquents at a reform school. He hoped that these large homogeneous groups could serve as contrast groups for researchers all over the country, who could compare their results with those in his data bank. He envisaged this bank as a kind of national resource which would make it unnecessary for each investigator to recruit his own contrast group.

I was pleased when he asked me if we would consider including our data on obese men in his bank, and I assured him that we would be glad to do so. We parted with an agreement to stay in touch and to do what we could to increase the usefulness of psychological tests.

Shortly afterwards other interests led Timothy Leary from the field of psychological testing. I also left soon thereafter, persuaded by the results of the study of obese men. After months of examining the data from every possible vantage point, the results were clear-cut and negative. The obese men showed no distinctive personality features. Many of them showed signs of emotional disturbance, but just as many non-obese men showed the same signs.

About that time I came across a remarkably similar study of obese women in a psychology journal. Its results were the same as ours. Psychological tests showed little difference between obese and non-obese women. There was good reason to give up on this line of research and to conclude that there are no psychological differences between the obese and the non-obese. But I had not completely given up hope of pursuing that quest. Perhaps, with a larger number of subjects. . . .

The opportunity was provided by what became known as the "Midtown Study." The first step in the study had been to identify a population of 110,000 persons consisting of everyone between the ages of 20 and 60 living in a specific area on the East Side of Manhattan. The area had been selected in order to include a wide variety of social and ethnic backgrounds. It included groups from the very lowest socio-economic status—unemployed people and those living in poverty, old lower-class ethnic neighborhoods, some middle-class areas, and a section of Park Avenue with some of the most expensive housing in the city. Altogether it included seven different ethnic groups, divided about equally into those who were foreign-born themselves, those with foreign-born parents, and those whose families had been in the United States for more than one generation. It was, in short, a microcosm of the city.

The 1660 subjects, representative of the 110,000, were selected for the study and interviewed in their homes by trained field workers for periods of two hours. The interviewers gathered information about the social class and ethnic background of the subjects, about the number of physical illnesses, and about a number of psychological factors. The researchers then scored each subject on a variety of indices of neurosis: "childhood anxiety, withdrawal, neurasthenia, depression, anxiety, rigidity, suspiciousness, and immaturity."

Although they had collected the weights of the subjects and entered them on IBM cards, the researchers, preoccupied with the more pressing issues of mental illness, had not done anything with them. They were just sitting there waiting for us. And the information was perfect for answering our question. From the heights and weights of the subjects we could calculate the percent overweight of each and identify those who were obese. For each obese and non-obese person there were indices of their psychological functioning. It was a simple matter to determine whether the obese persons were more or less neurotic than the non-obese.

The answer, when it finally came after all these years, was an anticlimax. The results were straightforward enough. Obese people were clearly more neurotic than non-obese people. In seven out of eight of the psychological measures they showed higher levels of neurosis. And this was true for men and women, young and old, and for all three social classes —low, middle and upper.

The problem was that the differences were really very small. Although they were statistically significant, largely because they were based on such a large sample, they were quite insignificant from a practical point of view.

Among obese people 63 percent showed immaturity, compared to 49 percent for the non-obese; for suspiciousness the comparable figures were 43 percent and 25 percent; for rigidity, 67 percent and 45 percent; for depression, 25 percent and 18 percent.

So finally the question was answered. And, as I had half-expected, the answer brought with it no great insights nor any prescription for action. From now on we could feel secure in talking about the greater amount of neurosis among obese people. But it was not at all clear how this related to their obesity, nor what was to be done about it. In a negative sense we had perhaps contributed something: it would be difficult to find in these data much support for the theory that neurosis was the cause of obesity.

As weeks went by the study kept bothering me, much like the original question had. It wasn't clear what more could be made of the results, but I had a strong conviction that somehow something more could be done with them.

The solution came one day, when, in a kind of reverie I found myself thinking about the correlation between social class and mental illness, which earlier investigators had discovered and which the Midtown Study had confirmed. My thoughts continued on to a similar correlation which we had found between social class and obesity. Suddenly it occurred to me that I had never heard any mention of such a correlation any place else. And yet, if my memory was correct, the differences had been enormous.

I could hardly wait to look at the data. And when I did, the results were stunning. No one had ever before noted a relationship between social class and obesity, and here it was— the most powerful influence we had ever looked at, perhaps the most powerful influence we would ever find.

In the ensuing months we analyzed and re-analyzed the data, exploring the relationship between all kinds of social factors and obesity. Hardly a week went by without some fascinating new finding. Furthermore, the discoveries fell into a general pattern, which became clearer the further we went. It seemed that the nearer a group of people approached the standards of upper-class values, the less the amount of obesity.

A great deal of what we learned was summarized in a graph which showed the relationship of socio-economic status to obesity among women. When the women's own socio-economic status was considered, there was a six-fold difference between those of lower and upper status. Obesity occurred in 30 percent of women of lower socio-economic status, in 16 percent of those in the middle status, and in only 5 percent of the upper status.

The data also allowed us to look at the socioeconomic status of the parents of our subjects, to determine whether social class influenced obesity, or vice versa. The results showed that the influence went both ways, but that social class had a far stronger influence upon obesity than obesity did upon social class. This conclusion is seen clearly in the graph, where the relationship of the parents' social class to the subject's obesity is almost as strong as that of the subject's own social class. Since the subject's obesity presumably could not have influenced the parents' social class, their social class must have influenced the obesity.

Nonetheless, obesity did influence social class to some degree. Another way of arranging the data shows this influence clearly. We divided our population into those people who remained in the social class into which they had been born, and those who either rose or fell in social class. Of the women who remained in the social class into which they were born, 17 percent were obese. Among women who moved downwards in social status, on the other hand, there was a higher fre-

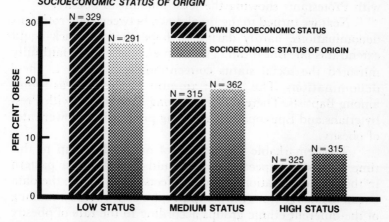

PREVALENCE OF OBESITY AMONG WOMEN
BY OWN SOCIOECONOMIC STATUS AND
SOCIOECONOMIC STATUS OF ORIGIN

quency of obesity—22 percent. Among those who moved up-wards in social class, the frequency of obesity fell to only 12 percent.

What does this mean? Does a subtle, or not so subtle discrimination against obese women result in their attracting only lower-status husbands and finding only lower-status jobs? Does it mean that those women who conform to upper-class standards—which prominently include thinness—are rewarded by higher-status husbands and higher-status jobs? It appears so, and others have since reported more direct evidence.

Exploring the relationship of social class to obesity was only the first of our analyses. We also examined the relationship between the number of generations during which a subject's family had been in the United States and the frequency of obesity. Twenty-four percent of foreign-born women were obese, and this percentage fell steadily with the number of generations in the United States, to a figure of 5 percent for women with no foreign-born grandparents.

We then looked at the breakdown of obesity according to religion. Starting with the three major religions, we determined the frequency of obesity among Protestants, Catholics, and Jews. By this time we were not surprised by the highly significant differences, nor by the nature of the differences. Obesity was most common among Jews, followed by Catholics, with Protestants showing the least amount of obesity.

Next we turned to the breakdown between the Protestant denominations, hardly daring to hope that our luck could extend this far. But it did. The frequency of obesity faithfully mirrored the social status conventionally ascribed to these denominations. The largest amount of obesity was found among Baptists. There was less among Methodists, with Presbyterians and Episcopalians showing progressively lower rates of obesity.

The remarkable consistency of our findings up to this time led us to expect that we could also detect a pattern in the ethnic affiliations of our subjects. Long before the data began to emerge from the computer, we constructed a ranking of the different ethnic groups according to the rate of obesity which we expected. The lowest frequency, clearly, would be among subjects whose families had been in the United States for a long period of time. Thereafter we guessed that the frequency of obesity would rise steadily as we moved eastward across Europe, starting with Great Britain. Ireland, we guessed would probably show a somewhat higher rate of obesity than Great Britain, and would then be followed, in turn, by Germany, Italy, Czechoslovakia, Hungary, and a Polish-Russian group. And that was how it turned out. Only one ethnic group was out of line. Among the Czechs, for some still unaccountable reason, a surprising 34 percent were obese, the highest rate among any of the groups.

six
Disturbance in the Body Image

By "disturbance in the body image" I mean the distorted picture that a person may have of the physical appearance of his own body. Such disturbances have long been known to occur in certain kinds of emotional disorders—from the chronic complaining of a paranoid individual about the size of his nose, to the delusions of severely depressed people about their bowels rotting away, and the schizophrenic patient's panicky sense that his body is disappearing. But we were slow to realize that the complaints of obese people about their bodies might be a form of disturbance in body image.

It certainly took me a long time. On the face of it, there was nothing unrealistic about the complaints of many obese people. Their bodies *were* huge, awkward and ungainly. And it wasn't until the study of "Obesity in Men"—the vain effort to save my Army contract—that an unexpected finding directed my attention to the phenomenon.

I had already observed that the intensity of obese people's dissatisfaction with their bodies varied widely, and not always in keeping with the extent of their obesity. Some of the bitterest complaints came from people, predominantly women, who were only moderately overweight, while far more obese people would seem to take a more tolerant and philosophical view of their affliction. I saw no consistent pattern, and in its absence I tended to view the self-censure as a more or less realistic response to a distressing situation.

What changed my mind was a paper which argued that efforts at weight reduction were less successful among adults who had been obese as children than they were among those who had developed their obesity in adult life. The idea was intriguing, and we proceeded to examine all of our subjects from this point of view. Sure enough, there was such a pattern.

Not only were the "childhood-onset obese" less successful in losing weight, they also tended to be more obese and more emotionally disturbed. Despite the fact that we examined only 25 men in this study (of which 12 were "childhood-onset obese" and 13 "adult-onset obese"), the distinction between the two groups was striking. Even in conversation, they differed. The childhood-onset obese seemed more emotionally labile, more complaining, more discouraged, more demanding. The adult-onset obese seemed more stable, more laconic, more matter-of-fact. We pursued these differences further.

Not one of the adult-onset obese men made any more than casual, realistic comments about his body. Among the childhood-onset obese men, on the other hand, 7 out of 12 complained about their bodies in extravagant and derogatory ways. Some childhood-onset obese did not complain about their bodies. But when a body image disturbance was found, it was always in a childhood-onset obese person.

Clearly disturbances in the body image of obese people represented a distinct phenomenon. Clearly it was the source of untold suffering. I decided to study it, and the one who taught me more than any other was Herbert Marx.

When he first came to see me, Herbert Marx was 21 years old, just entering his senior year of college . . . and thoroughly miserable. He was a short (5'6"), awkward young man, who walked slowly into the office, leaning backwards just a little—like a pregnant woman balancing her swollen abdomen. The folds of a double chin lay beneath what seemed a small head and youthful face, with no trace of beard on his smooth, pink cheeks. He weighed 205 pounds and was gaining rapidly.

Throughout our first meeting, in fact for a long time thereafter, Herbert seemed extraordinarily ill at ease, smiling too quickly, nodding agreement at the slightest opportunity. When he left the office at the end of our first meeting, he spoke in a manner clearly calculated to reassure me: "Well, doctor, I'm sure that we'll be finding out some very interesting things together." A perhaps modest understatement, but one which would prove prophetic.

As befitted someone who had had previous experience with psychiatric treatment, Herbert had come to our first meeting with a precise formulation of three "problems" for which he wanted help: "inconsistency, unpredictability, and going to extremes."

In talking about the first of these, he spoke in a small voice of muffled desperation. "I'm a Jekyll-Hyde character. I am somebody who can change completely within an hour. Just take, for example, a time when I might be reducing. Everything's going well. I'm trying to be with other people and doing everything that's right. Then, within a few minutes I just begin to eat, and I eat and eat and eat. And what do I eat? Only the denied foods." Seeing my puzzled expression, he explained, "Candy and pie, things like that. But that's not all. When I do this, I want to be completely alone. I feel ashamed of myself, like I have a dirty, dark secret.

"Then there's the unpredictability. I just don't have any idea when these changes are going to happen. I was living downtown this year, away from home, and for a while everything at school was going well. Then I suddenly began to eat. I fight with myself. I call myself a fat freak. I do everything I can to stop eating, but nothing works and I always end up eating.

"On top of that, I'm always going to extremes. Everything is always a hundred percent good or a hundred percent bad. There's no middle ground for me. I'm either dieting a hundred percent or gorging a hundred percent. If I break my diet, even just a little bit, then I figure that the whole day's ruined. And I feel so terrible that I curse myself mercilessly, but I go right on eating. It's gotten so this thing dominates my whole life. If I feel slighted, I don't think like other people do, 'Well, it's because I'm Jewish,' but only that I'm overweight. It's something that I can't fight back about, because I agree with people—I think that I should be despised for looking the way I do." And with a despairing sigh, he nervously motioned to his body.

As I sat listening to Herbert's barrage of self-derogation, I began to grow uneasy. I tried to slow the onslaught by asking some questions. What, for example, did he hope to get out of treatment. With that, he sat back and relaxed for the first time, and his speech, when it came, was slower and less convulsed.

"I guess I would just like to feel free and easy—not feel inferior, not always feel like I'm an outsider." But the respite was only temporary. He was soon talking about his weight again, and how he divided the whole world up into two classes, fat people and thin people. "I can't really say that I want to feel free and easy, unless I lose weight, because I worry all the time about what would happen if I weren't worrying about my weight. I mean what would happen if I didn't feel that everyone hated me? I don't know, but I guess I think I would just stop trying completely, and never stop eating and just swell up until I burst. No, it's not feeling free and easy that I want; it's getting down to 160 pounds."

It was some time before I discovered the full significance of Herbert Marx's goal of 160 pounds, since our weekly meetings were dominated by more immediate concerns. He began the third visit by arriving late, in a visibly distraught state, and launching quickly into a tormented stream of complaints. "I was good until yesterday, really I was. And then suddenly I developed the urge to over-eat—starches, candy, pie, all of the forbidden foods . . . you name it. So now my perfect record's smashed, completely shattered. And today is ruined —ruined as a perfect day, that is. So now I feel it should be a completely rotten day.

"I can't tell you how it started. I was good until after lunch yesterday. Then I went to my aunt's house, and I didn't find anyone there and got to wondering what was in the refrigerator. I kept arguing back and forth with myself and I finally ended up saying, 'You'd better get as much as you can now, before you get in control of yourself again. Here's your chance. Eat! Eat!'

"I don't know why I do all this. I'm terrified of being condemned by people for my weight. And yet of course they should condemn me. It's a despicable thing to weigh as much as I do. I'm grotesque and everyone's against me because of it. What do I have to offer anyway? A fat man. Everybody rejects me. I can tell at school they feel I'm not only fat but a greasy grind. All I can do is get good marks . . . The only hope is to get to 160."

He had tried going to the gym to play badminton during the struggle between "being good and being bad." But it had been hopeless. "I would have had to shower with all the other people, and then they would have made fun of me. And I couldn't leave to take a shower in my room, because it would have meant asking the gym teacher for permission. I hate gym teachers, and I don't ask favors of people I hate. I hate all athletes. They're jocks and I hate all jocks . . . But 160 is the magic number. If I can get there, I'll be able to shower with anyone."

He finally stopped long enough for me to ask him what weighing 160 pounds meant. He seemed genuinely surprised. "Why that was what I weighed when I had a date. I even went swimming then . . . twice."

Eventually I was able to piece together an account of Herbert Marx's weight over the years, with all its wild fluctuations, from his obese childhood and infancy, through countless successful and unsuccessful attempts at weight reduction. In all of this account the golden period had been his third year in high school, when he was 16 and weighed 160 pounds and had a date. But it had been followed by "that terrible summer," when he had started on a period of weight gain which had continued without interruption until he had reached 260 pounds.

The years before we began treatment had been characterized by increasingly rapid fluctuations in his weight. He had undergone psychotherapy the preceding year and spoke blandly of how much he had learned in the course of this treatment: "But it didn't seem to help my weight. I was 180 when I started with Dr. Wilson in the fall and 250 when I finished with him in the spring. But I don't blame him for that."

What did he blame for it? "At that time I thought, 'Well, I'm in treatment and sooner or later I'll get to the cause of my obesity. So in the meantime I'll just go ahead and eat whatever I want to and put the blame on the treatment.' Then after I stopped treatment I went on a very strict diet. It only took me seven months to get back down to 180. Then all of my good intentions just gave out." By the time Herbert Marx came to me, his eating had once again gotten out of control, his weight had risen to 205 pounds and showed no signs of stopping.

During the first months of treatment, I was able to learn something about Herbert Marx's family background. His parents had come from small Jewish communities in Eastern Europe while still children, had married young, and had soon settled into lives of bitter mutual recrimination. Much of the animosity centered around Herbert's father's occupation as a junk dealer. With increasing acidity, Mrs. Marx assailed her husband for his incompetence and his inability to "get ahead in life." She was joined in her assaults by two sisters who lived close by. Together these women dominated their extended family. Although frequently bickering among themselves, they presented a solid front toward the rest of the family—often demeaning and invariably hostile.

When Herbert's family moved to a new neighborhood and his father was unable to get a new job, the full fury of the three sisters was unleashed. And one day, when Herb was 14 years old, his father just disappeared. He never saw him again. There was just one wistful reminder: each week, without fail, there arrived at the doorstep two or three recent editions of magazines addressed to "the Marx family" in his father's handwriting, with no return address.

Not long after the disappearance of his father, Herbert's mother found a small house with an apartment upstairs and a candy store and newsstand below. And as the details of his life unfolded, I could scarcely believe the degree to which his background paralleled that of Hyman Cohen.

"Mother works extremely long hours in the store—from seven in the morning until ten at night. It's terribly hard work . . . There is a great deal of petty thievery and the customers are very hard to please. I used to help out in the store on weekends, and it was usually a mess. Mother and I were always fighting. I really don't know what we were fighting about. All I know is that there's just a lot of tension around her all the time, and I was always stealing candy and ice cream and eating it.

"I never liked the store. I always felt that it was just a petty little business, that it wasn't nice. I was always worrying about people stealing things, and I just hated the whole business. I hated it." And caught in the ugly memory, he shuddered.

About two months after the start of treatment, Herbert Marx's complaints and self-derogation began to dry up. He talked more and more often about how good he was feeling and of his hopes for the future. "I'm better, much better. I'm really doing things that I never thought I could do. Like today I left the potatoes and meat on my plate. Before, I used to feel a terrible drive to eat. Now there's hardly any drive at all.

"I even ran for the train today, and it's the first time I've done that in ages. I think it's a symbol. I used to say

to myself that it would make me look like a fat fool to run.
And I'd rationalize that I probably wouldn't be able to make
the train anyway. So I'd say to myself, 'Why not wait around
till the next train and feel miserable?'

"But it's different now. Don't you notice anything unusual about me today? . . . I'm wearing my contact lenses.
I got them last year but I never got up the initiative to use
them. I figured nobody would notice. But I started wearing
them over the weekend and I've worn them every day since
then. What do you think?"

As the weeks went by, Herbert's weight fell, from 205
to 180, and his confidence rose. "I've passed the halfway mark
on the road to 160. I know I might be wrong, but I just have
this conviction that the only way people think about me is
in terms of my weight. When I get below 160 I'll be very
nearly perfect. And I just can't imagine anyone criticizing
me or not liking me then. Of course, I might find that people
will hate me because I'm Jewish, or because I'm a greasy
grind and get good marks. But right now I feel that everyone
will have to like me. It's inevitable."

The honeymoon phase of treatment was now in full swing.
It had been gratifying, very gratifying in fact, to watch the
change in this morose and hopelessly discouraged young man,
to watch the growth of hope and the rise in his self-esteem.
And somehow, despite his euphoria, I didn't feel as concerned
as I might have over an impending depression. Perhaps it
was because he soon began to use his new-found confidence
to try to achieve a long deferred goal.

"Now I'm all set for the next step. Now I want to have
a date. That's my next project. So I'm driving to 160. The
pressure is on to get there. I know it's irrational, but that's
what I weighed when I had the date in high school."

What had happened on that date, I wondered. It had
seemed to mean so much to him. Why wasn't there a second
one? "Basically, I guess, it was because Mother disapproved.
She was waiting for me when I came back from the date
and asked me what we had done, so I told her. We sat in
Gladys' living room and talked. That was all. But Mother

said, 'That isn't what you do on a date. You take the girl out to a movie or something.' Anyhow, she disapproved, and I lost my ambition. And my weight went up again and I never had another date, never . . .' "

But Herbert Marx was determined to change that. Right after mid-year exams, he got a job waiting on tables in a local restaurant two or three nights a week, in order to have a small fund ready for dating expenses. His mother expressed concern that this work might detract from his studies, but he reassured her with ease. And three months after starting treatment his weight had fallen to 173 pounds.

"I'm pulling out the stops. I know my goals. One hundred and sixty pounds and then a date. I say to myself, 'Let's get there. Don't let anything stand in the way.' "

He left the office looking radiant.

He did not appear for his next appointment, or the one after that. He didn't call; he didn't write. He just disappeared. So I wrote him, asking if anything had gone wrong, saying that I would like to hear from him. He didn't reply. Then, a month after his last visit, he called to make an appointment.

I was stunned to see Herbert as he walked slowly down the hall to my office, 25 pounds heavier. Bloated and bitter, he slunk into a chair and gazed at the floor. He began in a low voice, "I've been eating like a pig . . ."

Laboriously, over the next month, we pieced together the story of what had gone wrong. At first Herbert said he thought it was a matter of "simple overconfidence," as he called it. "I got to feeling so cocky about things, and I said to myself, 'Why waste your money on Dr. Stunkard? He is sincere, but you don't need him. It just kills an afternoon when you could be studying. . . .' Then I wished I had my old doctor, Dr. Wilson, someone who knew my case. I had the feeling, 'You're not qualified. You don't know enough about my case.' And then I started eating, and I didn't want you to interfere with it. When I got on a binge, nothing else mattered. 'To hell with reason . . . to hell with Dr. Stunkard . . . to hell with me. I just want to get that chocolate sundae into my belly.' "

It took another month to disentangle the issues. Over-eating had started immediately after Herbert had received his mid-year grades. Although he had earned, as usual, honor grades in most of his courses, he had received a C in one. Naturally it had been disappointing, but it seemed an inade-quate explanation for the remarkable reversal of his upward course. We puzzled over this question for quite a while. Then, almost gratuitously, Herbert remarked that he had called his mother the evening his grades had come out.

Her reaction had been disappointment, then outrage. How did Herbert dare to bring her this kind of grade after all that she had done for him? Was this her reward for the long hours in the candy store? This showed how right she had been about his not taking the job waiting on tables. That would have to stop.

"I just couldn't convince her that that wasn't the way things were, that the work that they based the grades on was all finished before I took the job. She just kept harping on the job, so I had to tell her I would quit it." His first binges began the next morning. Was it the grade or was it his mother's reaction which had been the agent of this change? Neither. The cause was his giving in to his mother and once again becoming her little boy.

During the next six months, plagued by incessant and recurrent eating binges, Herbert gained 50 more pounds. "It's perverse. I'm not eating just to fill my stomach, but to get in as many calories as I can. It's a furious race to see how much I can eat in how short a time. I don't over-eat the way somebody else might. It's repulsive. I'm just gorging, panting, having a bowel movement. Afterwards I feel terribly guilty and unbearably thirsty . . . an incredible thirst."

This bright and articulate young man, driven by depres-sion, told me more about disturbances in body image than I had heard from all other sources up to that time. The linkage with depression seemed critical. During the initial three months, which had been characterized by growing euphoria, Herbert had spoken progressively less about his dissatisfaction with his body. Now, immersed in depression, he could talk of little else. By the time he returned to treatment these concerns had already acquired an almost delusional character.

"Yesterday when I was in the store trying to get some special graph paper, the sales lady said they didn't have it, even though I knew they did." He stopped and nodded with a significant look. I frowned, quizzically, and he explained, "Don't you see—she was so overwhelmed by my appearance that she couldn't think straight. She couldn't even remember what they had in stock."

The distortions didn't end there. Early in this new period of depression Herbert began to withdraw from his friends. "It just isn't fair for me to be around them. Like Jerome—he has a terrible time because he's associated with me. I've ruined his reputation; it's like being associated with a gangster."

All hopes of dating dissolved. "How can I go out with a girl, any girl? She'll hate me for being fat and mentally ill." Puzzled, I asked about the nature of this mental illness. "Obsessive-compulsive. I've been reading about it in medical books, and I know what it is."

I shook my head and smiled at Herbert and said, "You dope," in what must have been an affectionate way. He brightened for a moment and sat forward and smiled. Then he sighed and said, "But that's just your reaction, and you're paid to deal with it. You'll find that the general public isn't so tolerant of mental illness."

Nor, he was convinced, were they tolerant of bodies such as his. He kept having recurring hopes of being able to go swimming, in order to expend the calories he was now consuming so avidly. "But how can I do it? I can't let anyone see me in the nude. They would just hate me. And they would have every justification for hating me, because they would see everything I hate about myself—this (with an expression of horrified disdain) obese body of mine."

As the months went by, these hateful preoccupations with his body assumed a more and more central role in Herbert Marx's life. It was as if he felt that nothing ever happened to him except in some kind of (usually derogatory) relationship to his body. And the last remaining shreds of self-confidence

were periodically shattered by experiences which reminded
him of his weight. On one occasion, for example, he had
screwed up the courage to ask some friends to go to the movies
with him. On his way to meet them at the theater he passed
a large plate-glass window of a downtown department store,
and suddenly caught a glimpse of himself in it. "I was just
stunned by it. I felt such loathing and hatred toward myself
that I turned around and went home. I couldn't face anyone
after an experience like that."

This was the first of a number of times that seeing himself
in a store window precipitated such a reaction. "It's gotten
so that even when I'm feeling well, just looking at myself
in a store window makes me sick. It's gotten so that I'm very
careful not to look by accident. It's a feeling that people have
a right to hate me and to hate anyone who looks as fat as
me. As soon as I see myself, I feel an uncontrollable burst
of hatred. I just look at myself and say, 'I hate you! You're
loathsome, disgusting, despicable.' "

These reactions to his own image in a mirror seemed
so striking and so predictable that in our research on disturbances in body image, we began to ask obese people how
they felt when they looked at themselves in the mirror. The
answers to this simple question were frequently as helpful
as any other measure in assessing the presence and intensity
of disturbances in body image. Some very obese people could
look at themselves in the mirror and quite matter-of-factly
describe what they saw, without any particular emotional
reaction. For others, like Herbert Marx, the intensity of the
disorder increased with the intensity of the depression.

I will never forget the first time that I asked Herbert
to look into the mirror in my office. The mirror was so high
on the wall that it was necessary for him to stand on his
chair in order to see himself. After a long pause he said, "Well,
there it is. And I guess I don't feel so bad about it. I feel
more detached."

Encouraged, I asked if he felt that I hated him for this
body which he now saw reflected. "No, I don't think so. I
wonder if my feelings don't have to do with the person that's

with me. You're with me and I feel all right. But if Mother was with me, I'd feel sick to my stomach. Sometimes I might have forgotten for a few minutes that I was fat, and then, all of a sudden, I'd remind myself: 'You're fat, boy, and don't you ever forget it!' It's like a brand you wear. . . ."

"And what about when you're alone?" I asked.

"It's bad then," he replied. "Almost as bad as if I was with Mother. It's funny, but I think it depends on whether I'm with someone I trust. And when I'm alone, it's like I'm with people I don't trust."

The intensity of the disturbance in body image was influenced not only by the person he was with, but also by his emotions, often with startling immediacy. This was particularly clear during the period of intense guilt which followed an eating binge. "It was really uncanny last Saturday after the binge. Beforehand people looked all right to me. They seemed friendly enough, or at least neutral. And then within ten minutes everything changed. They all began to look vicious. Everyone I saw was a threat to me. Everyone. And everyone hated me."

Some psychiatrists believe that depression consists of two separable components—helplessness and hopelessness. This distinction seemed useful in considering Herbert Marx's depression, for it seemed to involve a far greater measure of helplessness than of hopelessness. At times his description of these feelings achieved a poetic quality: "I feel that I have no direction any more, no purpose . . . I'm like a feather blowing in the wind . . . a chip of wood floating down a river. A worthless cipher . . . I have no idea what to do when I finish work at the end of the day and no idea of where to go. So I just go to my room and lie down, or else I go out and eat . . . I'm completely directionless. I can't be sure of anything any more. I don't know what I believe.

"I'm empty . . .There's nothing there. I'm just like a shadow walking around the laboratory. When I'm driving the car, it's like there's no one behind the wheel. It's not that I don't know where I'm driving to, it's just that I don't know why. I feel like going up to people and asking them what their secret is, how they know to do what they're doing. It's very lonely and very frightening."

These dark moods of helplessness were rarely paralleled by comparable feelings of hopelessness. Often the depression was punctuated by brief but fierce periods of asceticism. He would embark upon rigidly restrictive 600- and 800-Calorie diets and snarl between clenched teeth, "What I need is *real discipline*. That gym instructor was right. He should have *made* me take a shower with the others, and made me so damned embarrassed that I wouldn't eat for weeks."

And when I kept raising the possibility that he might achieve at least a measure of happiness without weighing 160 pounds, he would counter vigorously, "No, absolutely no. No possibility! I'm a criminal by being over-weight. There is absolutely no chance of being happy. I am *just not allowed* to be happy while I'm overweight. If I were happy while I was overweight, the foundations of my whole world would be shaken."

Despite the severity of Herbert Marx's depression, and despite his weight gain, I somehow felt that matters were going to improve. Perhaps I was buoyed by his reaction to our visits. "I usually wake up feeling fine on the days when I am going to come in here. And I usually feel pretty good all day and for a few hours after I see you. But then the troubles begin again."

This kind of responsiveness led me to believe that he was not as sunken into depression as he sometimes appeared to be. And I was encouraged one day at the end of a particularly lugubrious hour, when he stopped at the door, turned and said in a faint, pleading voice, "Don't let me stop treatment, Doctor, no matter how much I try."

So we continued. And the weeks went by, with Herbert complaining about his failures and inadequacies. Gradually, when these pressures abated, we were able to return to the circumstances which seemed to be perpetuating his difficulties. We examined his eating binges in as much detail as possible, paying particular attention to the circumstances which seemed to trigger them. There, in the kind of conflict which preceded a binge, we began to see the problems which pervaded Herbert's life. And, as he grew more aware, the binges themselves lost some of their frightening quality, and became vehicles for mastery.

For a long time the common elements that precipitated binges remained obscure. But eventually the insights began to come. As with Hyman Cohen, it began to appear that a period of intense discomfort preceded the binge; and also like Hyman Cohen, there were hints that Herbert's discomfort was related to feelings of having been taken advantage of and of not being true to himself.

Whatever the reason, when his weight had reached 225 pounds, it began to level off. And the intensity of his complaints began to slacken. Periods of well-being began to recur, and during them he returned to his old preoccupation with dating. Eventually he hit upon an ingenious strategy. Since he couldn't stand having a girl look at him, he decided to establish a relationship by mail. He backed and filled for a few weeks on this project, and then finally sent a latter to Gladys, the girl with whom he had had the only date of his life, almost six years before.

The following week Herbert arrived at my office exuberant. Gladys had replied with a long, friendly letter. He responded immediately, and since then had written her every day. I was pleased by this turn of events, but felt the poignancy of what was happening. "One thing that makes me feel very reassured about Gladys is that she has taken a course in abnormal psychology. That makes me more confident that she can understand me."

As might have been expected, the correspondence with Gladys marked the end of Herbert Marx's downhill course. During the next five months his depression lifted, he lost 30 pounds, and there was less and less talk about his body. When he did speak about it, it was with far less vehemence and disdain.

Early in his writing relationship with Gladys, he had worried about his "dishonesty."

"Dishonesty?" I asked.

"I'm 70 pounds heavier than she remembers me. It's dishonest not to let her know. I've just got to tell her," he explained. I said that it might or might not be dishonest not to let her know, but that if he felt he had to tell Gladys about his weight, he should go ahead, and should also tell her how he himself felt about it. When he finally did, she wrote back at once telling him she understood.

Then she began signing her letters "fondly" instead of "yours truly." He kept wondering about this. What did it mean? He began to feel that he simply had to go ahead and see her. It didn't seem quite so impossible as before. "Until you mentioned it to me, Dr. Stunkard, it just had never occurred to me that her writing might mean that she cared about me. I just thought she was interested in writing me because she had taken abnormal psychology. But you're right. Signing her letters 'fondly' must mean something." And he beamed.

As the derogatory comments about his body lessened, Herbert Marx began to do things which he had longed to do for years. Sitting down and crossing his legs he held up one foot. "See what I'm wearing? My white bucks. I've had them for over a year but never wore them for fear of looking ridiculous. And now I'm wearing them even though I weigh more than 200 pounds. That's a real victory. Just like not having to wear a sweater." And I noticed that for the first time since I had known him, Herb was in shirtsleeves. "I don't need the camouflage any more."

Even the feelings of helplessness disappeared. "I feel like I'm the boss now. I'm doing what I want to do. Almost every decision about my life is one that I make. It's an entirely different ball game."

But the matter of Gladys was still unresolved. For three months their correspondence continued, she making no moves to see him, and he still afraid to risk it. By keeping to our discussions on the topic, I was able to induce Herb to explore the remaining fears which kept him from seeing her. There were some that he couldn't even write about to her. "I don't even know what I'm supposed to do on a date. Damn it all, why can't I tell her that I'm scared to see her, that I've thought for years that women hate fat men?" And, "I always thought that if someone went out with a girl, all of his loyalty would be due to her and he couldn't do anything without her. That's how I felt, that I would have to be sort of enslaved to her and give her all my time. Like the way I feel about Mother."

Quietly, by simply not allowing our conversation to diverge very long from this issue, I kept Herb talking about a date. His confidence rose. And finally there came the day when he entered the office, sat down and grinned irrepressibly. "Well, I saw her.

"And as soon as she saw me she said, 'You certainly do exaggerate.' I knew she was talking about my weight. I was just amazed at how understanding she was. And you're right, it wasn't just because she had taken abnormal psychology."

I was particularly pleased by the nature of Herbert's sense of well-being. When I asked him about "feeling so good," he corrected me. "It isn't that I'm feeling 'so good,' it's just that I'm not feeling bad any more. It isn't like that time last fall, when I was driving towards 160 and feeling so high about it. Still, you know, I'm amazed at myself. You know the L&M advertising slogan, 'They said it couldn't be done'? Well, I keep saying that to myself, and then I add: 'But I've done it, I've gone and done it.' "

These feelings of accomplishment were mirrored in his activities. "I went swimming yesterday, and it wasn't too hard. I did feel a little scared when I went to the gym, but that was nothing compared to the feeling of success I had later. I guess I felt sort of uneasy when I thought of people looking at me. But then I just got the feeling, 'If they don't like how I look, to hell with them!' It was terrific."

Herbert's weight began to melt away. He lost nearly seven pounds in the week after he saw Gladys, and the weight loss seemed different from his other efforts. "Now I just don't have any impulse to eat. Before, I used to match my drive to reduce against the drive to eat. But it's not the same now—I don't have *either* kind of drive. There's just no desire to eat."

I asked what had brought about the change, and he replied, "I feel like I'm in control of my life . . . I seem to have more respect for myself. I feel that at least one person really cares, and believes that I'm worthwhile. You pointed that out. Gladys must care for me if she would spend so much time writing letters."

The first date with Gladys had taken place in the middle of October, a year after Herbert had started treatment. He actually saw her only three times during the following month, but each of the dates seemed to go well, and he returned from them happy and confirmed in his more tolerant views of his body. "When I was with her last time I even forgot that I was overweight. I just walked along so nonchalant and natural that I wouldn't have known myself in the old days."

Unfortunately, this happy state of affairs was not to last long. By the beginning of December, Herbert began to report eating binges, and his weight, which had fallen to 200 pounds, rose to 220 pounds within a month. At first the reasons for these developments were unclear. Then it gradually developed that Herbert had been having increasing difficulty in getting a date with Gladys. If he didn't call a long time before the date, he would find her busy; and with each rejection he found it more and more difficult to call.

After several such incidents, I urged Herbert to ask her if things were different. For a time he ignored this suggestion, but finally, after one particularly close therapy hour, he acceded. "O.K. I get the point. I'll find out what's happening, no matter how bad it is. Damn the torpedoes, full speed ahead!" And he shook my hand as he left the office that day, saying, "I always feel so much better when I go out of here."

The period of indecision and ambiguity was brought to a close just before the Christmas holidays. Herbert wrote Gladys a short, carefully composed letter asking if something had changed in their relationship. Her answer, when it came a few days later, had an electric, and strangely paradoxical effect.

Herbert came to the office in the afternoon, a few hours after having received her letter. He was smiling and said that he felt elated. He had been turned down by Gladys because she had become interested in another boy and wanted to go steady with him. She said that "it wasn't because I was fat but just a question of bad timing. She said she had met this other boy just before we started to go out."

He went on in a euphoric manner: "When I received the letter I went from darkest night to brightest sunshine. I went home right away and threw away all the food I had been hoarding for a binge this evening. I think I feel this way because of the relief over knowing that it is all down in black and white now. And also because she had said that it hadn't mattered that I was fat. I really feel grateful to her, because she just rejected me as a date. But she accepted me as a friend and as a human being. So I've started a new diet, and I'm going to start calling up some of the girls I met while I was dating Gladys."

I was surprised by this reaction, and not entirely reassured by it. It seemed to have much of the elation that had characterized the first honeymoon phase of our treatment. Unhappily, these reservations proved valid. The depression, which had begun tentatively and uncertainly during the period of uncertainty over his relations with Gladys, now struck with full force; and Herbert sank into a despair as pervasive as that of the previous spring. His over-eating raged out of control, and in three months his weight rose from 200 to 267 pounds.

Herbert's first response to the loss of Gladys was to return to his old, compulsive studying during every free hour of the day and night. He seemed to suffer extravagantly; and when we discussed the way he talked about this suffering, he conceded that he might have been embellishing it. But why? The answer, when it finally came, surprised me by its directness. "Mother always said, 'God will bless you for your suffering.' "

Not long after that Herb began to reexperience an intense hatred of his body. Knowing that this problem was likely to recur, we had been on the look-out for it and for its immediate determinants. And we discovered that those were neither the over-eating, which was already in full swing, nor his weight itself. Instead, the disturbance in body image was related to the loss of that feeling which had become so very important to him, the feeling of being in control of his own life.

Earlier, being in control of his life had meant regulating his eating. Now his hopes and his goals had expanded into more human dimensions; they included going out on dates and being relaxed with other people. The benefits which he had obtained from treatment now seemed almost perversely turned against him, for his expectations of himself were now so much greater.

Three weeks after Gladys' letter, Herbert reported the return of the disturbances in his body image. From the first, they were intense; and, if such were possible, his guilt about the binges was greater than ever. He found himself totally unable to eat in front of other people, and confined his eating, now in excessive spurts, almost entirely to his room. If he couldn't arrange to be there, he would take his food into the bathroom and lock himself in a stall to eat.

All kinds of casual events took on new meanings. "Today one of my friends waved at me from across the street. He's always been someone who has been nice to me, and so I couldn't read hatred into his wave. But I did feel that it was very sad." I asked Herbert what gave him that feeling, and in a thoroughly defeated voice he replied, "He's sad because he can feel my sadness."

As Herbert Marx's treatment moved into the second year, the reasons for his periods of weight loss and weight gain became clearer. The first period of weight loss seemed to have occurred almost automatically, in response to his hopes and illusions about treatment. The succeeding five months of weight gain had been triggered by what seemed an almost trivial incident, his C at mid-year, followed by his mother's using the grade to get him to quit his job. The next cycle of weight loss and weight gain seemed entirely dependent upon his acceptance and then rejection by Gladys.

Over the months Herbert was able to detach himself enough from the immediate pressures of outside events to consider the origins of his reactions, and the special meanings that certain experiences had for him. I was particularly interested in how his disturbance in body image had started, and how it had come to occupy such a prominent place in his life. I told him that I was baffled as to how anyone could so consistently disparage himself and his body, and could not understand how this disorder had come about. Eventually we found out.

Herbert was discussing a visit home shortly after Gladys' letter of rejection. He told how his mother had spent a great deal of time telling him about the visit of the child of a relative. "All she talked about was how little the child ate. She just went on and on about how it wouldn't eat. Finally I called her on this. I asked her what she was getting at. And then she told me. She said, 'I am sorry to have to say this to you, Herbert, but I hate all fat people and I always will.'

"I was stunned by this and she probably noticed, but she went right on. She said that everybody in the family hated fat people, they just *hated* them. She got all wound up about it and told me that the only reason she had ended up with a schlemiel like my father was because she was fat and nice men didn't want her. She said that she had weighed 160 pounds then, and that was bad enough, but it was nothing to what I looked like now.

"I got terribly upset, and then she told me that she prays night and day for me to be happy. That just made me feel more guilty. The only thing she wants in life is for me to be happy, and I'm not happy, so I'm letting her down."

I asked Herbert why he thought that he wasn't happy. "How can a person be happy when he's fat? I know that just as well as Mother does."

I didn't leave the matter there. How could his mother, I asked, be so solicitous of his happiness as to pray night and day for it, while at the same time hating all fat people? Wasn't this inconsistent? Herbert left the office that day, puzzling over this question.

To my surprise and pleasure, he went straight home with it. He reminded his mother about her statement that she hated all fat people and then asked her how this applied to him. Her response was prompt: "You, I love—all the rest, I hate." Then he raised the question of his unhappiness. Why did she think he was unhappy?

Apparently his mother answered, as if it were the most natural thing in the world, "Because it's impossible to be happy when you're fat." When Herbert told me this, I reminded him of similar sentiments coming from his lips not too long before. He frowned, and then nodded in agreement. Together we began to gather evidence to reconstruct the origins of his hatred for his body.

At times he would even solicit this evidence. "Over the weekend I decided to face her again. I went in and asked her to tell me again how she felt about fat people. She said that she couldn't help it, but that she just *hated* fat people. Then she got carried away. She said that fat people were pigs, and they ought to wear signs on their front and back saying 'I am a pig!' "

One Saturday evening Herbert and his mother had gone out to dinner, and things had gone well for a while. But as soon as the waiter had set down the butter, his mother reached over and grabbed it away. He felt disappointed, angry, and hurt, then soon afterwards, restless. ". . . And when we were walking home, Mother wanted to hold hands with me. This made me feel even worse. I don't want her to treat me like a date.

"I got away from her as soon as I could, and then I just found myself eating . . . all sorts of forbidden foods—candy, soda, ice cream, hot dogs. I hated every bite. It was nauseating, just an automatic gobbling down of the food and wanting to get out of there. I felt that I just *had* to do it. And I didn't enjoy it at all. It was like a nightmare. I felt furious at Mother. I kept thinking that she shouldn't have done it. I kept thinking about how she said fat people ought to wear signs on their front and back that say, 'I am a pig.' I just couldn't shake it loose. And it felt like everyone on the street was looking at me and was my enemy. So I slunk off home and went to bed. I hardly slept at all."

During this period when we were paying special attention to his mother, Herbert commented about her unhappiness and discouragement, epitomized by her old refrain: "I've no Mazel [luck] . . . The world's against me." These words, I remembered, were the same ones Herbert himself had used. I also remembered that, at the time he had used them, he hadn't seemed as hopeless as the phrases implied. Here, perhaps, was the reason—they were a kind of verbal behavior taken over from his mother and used to express unhappiness, but not the deeper despair which they suggested.

As we began to accumulate more and more evidence bearing upon the sources of his difficulties, Herbert threw himself into the search with increasing enthusiasm. It didn't seem to reduce the intensity of his depression, but we did learn more and more about the historical origins of his vulnerability. And in the course of our probings he became less vulnerable. I remember with pride the day that he came into the office with a firm, angry step and threw on my desk a letter he had received the previous day from his mother. It was a short note, telling him that he was a terrible disappointment to the people who loved him, and asking why didn't he appreciate their love?

Hers was a pathetic scrawl, and under other circumstances I might have pitied the agony behind it. But I was too busy glorying in Herb's response. "What the hell does she think she's doing, sending me letters like this? It's the same old game, and I'm through playing it. She can just go to hell with her love. That's what she can do with it."

It was hard to say why, but it seemed that just at this time, when Herbert was beginning to gain some understanding of how his upbringing had warped him, his mother and aunts escalated their complaints. It may simply have been their response to his continuing weight gain. But I began to wonder if, in some subtle manner, he was not beginning to convey to them his growing disinclination to play the part they had always assigned him. In any event, the assaults continued; and we studied them and learned how he had been hurt. And he began to talk about fighting back.

Liberation was not easy. If Herbert didn't respond to his mother's pleas, an aunt could be counted on to keep up the pressure. "Yesterday one of them said to me, 'If you could only see yourself as others do. You just don't know what you are doing to yourself.'" Herb pounded his hand on the table and said that he damned well did know what he was doing to himself, and why couldn't they let him alone? "If you can't like your own body, what can you like? I've always felt different and *bad*. They keep telling me I'm no good and I agree with them. They're always saying, 'You're just like your father.' And nothing could be worse than that. He's the devil in that family."

He was able to trace back to his family the genesis of some of the fears which were keeping him from dating after his break-up with Gladys. "I keep being afraid of what a girl would think about this feminized anatomy of mine—my big hips and chest. My aunt is always talking about it. She says, 'Your breasts are larger than a woman's,' and 'your stomach is fatter than a pregnant woman's.' You can imagine how that makes me feel. It makes me feel lower than a snake. But if I were to get infuriated and walk away, they would call me a coward and yell after me, 'The truth hurts' . . . and things like, 'See? He's running away . . . just like his father.' It makes me feel like I'm evil, the most terrible person that ever lived. I don't hang around and let them do that to me any more, but still that's the way I think about myself when I'm feeling badly."

As Herbert continued to recount the seemingly endless disparagements to which he had been subjected, I began to wonder how he had been able to control his resentment over the years. Why was it that he seldom showed any resentment of their constant battering? He explained it quite simply: "Until recently I always thought that they were right and I was wrong. And I guess I still do feel that way when I'm around them. It's just in here that I begin to think that maybe I'm not wrong all the time, and maybe they don't have the right to talk to me that way.

"They're always telling me, 'You're killing your mother,'

and I know how upset I can make her. I don't know whether
I really think I'm killing her or not; but it's all so frightening
that I guess I feel I should think whatever they tell me to
think. I don't know. . . ."

Not long afterwards, when he was telling me about further disparagements by his aunts, I asked him how this made
him feel. Suddenly the old tired mood was gone. He looked
angry, and he said, with an outraged intensity that I had
never before heard from him, "I'll never allow them to do
this to me again."

Less than two weeks later, Herbert put this promise into
action. It was early in the spring, at a family meeting at the
house of an aunt and uncle, where he was planning to spend
the summer. As far as he was concerned, the living arrangements had already been confirmed. During the course of the
evening, his uncle, who was somewhat of an outsider and
knew it, attempted to curry favor with his two sisters-in-law.
Announcing in a loud voice that Herbert's weight was just
too much for him to take, he went on to say that Herbert
couldn't live in their house unless he had lost 50 pounds by
June (only two months away).

"I felt very cold and very angry," Herbert reported in
icy tones. "I just said, 'Very well then, I'll find some place
else to live.' And I left the house, and for once in my life
I didn't feel bad."

Within a month Herb had screwed up his courage sufficiently to take on his aunts. The encounters were usually
brief and ugly, and were followed by long silences, or by an
attempt by one aunt to intervene on behalf of the other who
had been engaged in the latest conflict.

As Herbert approached independence from his mother
and aunts, I expected a period of dieting and weight loss.
But he lost little weight. The effects on his body image were,
therefore, thrown into bold relief. He still weighed 260 pounds
on the summer afternoon when, after telling me how he was
increasing his social life, he said, "You know, I don't seem
at all worried about my body any more. As I walk along
now, I feel as though I am very light on my feet. It's absurd,

I know, but it's almost as though I weigh 140 pounds." As the summer wore on, this feeling deepened. He began to wear Bermuda shorts and colorful sport clothes. Greatest of all triumphs, he went swimming. He had, in fact, reduced, but he still weighed 240 pounds when he said, "It's gotten so that I almost *feel* thin. It's a completely different way I feel about myself, and it doesn't have anything to do with how much I weigh. I feel that I'm in command now."

Gradually, over a period of years, he began to lose weight, and the remarkable freedom from concern with his body continued. Occasionally, following a particularly painful event (which was usually coupled with an eating binge), some of the old feelings would return. But in spite of weighing over 220 pounds for the next year and a half, his disparagement of his body seemed gone. "I just can't get over it. I feel so good. It's as if my mind says that I'm not overweight, but when I look at my body it says I still am. I said 'still' because it seems to me like a cultural lag that I'm still fat. I really ought to be thin now, and I will be in a while, and it surprises me to realize that I'm not."

After all the ups and downs of this treatment, with Herbert still weighing 20 pounds more than when he first had come to see me two and a half years before, I should have been skeptical of his optimism. Curiously enough, I wasn't. I had come to believe in this young man. And although I still didn't know how he was going to do it, I shared Herbert's confidence that he would lose the weight. What became of our prophecy is saved for the next chapter.

In the meantime, I would like to tell something of the systematic studies which complemented this more intensive study of one man. I thought I understood how Herbert's disorder had developed, something about the circumstances which alternately exacerbated and alleviated it, and, finally, how it might be successfully treated. But how common were such disturbances and how often were they so severe? Which of the circumstances that seemed to have caused Herbert's disorder were peculiar only to his difficulties and which were more general? Was the disorder ever relieved by weight reduction? And what about the provocative suggestion from the earlier study of 25 obese men that these disturbances were found only among people who had been obese since childhood?

With these questions in mind, my colleagues and I studied in some detail 74 obese people.

As we had suspected, body image disturbances did not occur in emotionally healthy obese people. In fact, we found them in only a minority of neurotic obese people. Seventeen of the 74 patients in our study showed severe body image disturbances—and all of these were people who had become obese during childhood or adolescence. It was clear that their disturbances in body image were different from those which occur in brain-damaged and schizophrenic people, or in normal people under the influence of drugs, hypnosis, and fatigue. They resembled instead the disturbances reported by people suffering from deformities of parts of their body, such as deformities of the face, breasts and genitals.

The main feature of the obese person's disturbance was the constant preoccupation with obesity, often to the exclusion of any other personal characteristic. It made no difference whether the person was talented, wealthy, or intelligent; his weight was his overriding concern, and he saw the entire world in terms of body weight. Such patients often divided society into people of differing weights, and then responded to them in terms of this division: envy toward anyone thinner and contempt for those who were fatter. At the center of this attitude was the appraisal of his own body as grotesque, even loathsome, and the feeling that others viewed it with only horror and contempt.

When body image disturbances did occur, their intensity fluctuated widely, even over short periods of time. When things were going well and a person with a body image disturbance was in good spirits, he was troubled little or not at all by his disability, although it was rarely far from awareness. Let things go badly, however, let a depressive mood ensue, and at once all of the derogatory and unpleasant things in his life would become focused on his obesity, and his body would become the explanation and symbol of his unhappiness.

Despite these short-term fluctuations in intensity, body image disturbances persisted with remarkably little change over long periods of time and in the face of wide variation in life's circumstances. Weight reduction, for example, appeared to have little effect upon the disturbance, a finding which surprised and dismayed a number of obese people. Neither the extent of the weight reduction nor its duration seemed able to correct the disturbance in body image. And I have yet to hear reports of spontaneous remission of the disorder.

We also discovered that the intense self-consciousness which Herbert Marx exhibited was commonplace among the patients with body image disturbances. Almost all of them, like Herbert, had serious difficulties in relationships with the opposite sex. One attractive young woman, who in other days would have been considered pleasingly plump, put her despair in dramatically succinct terms: "Who'd want to marry an elephant?" Another woman said that her body made her feel embarrassed with men whom she thought were "normal." "So I tend to pick up abnormal men. I tend to hang out with fairies. That way I don't feel I have to compete with real women."

As sad as these stories were, the study itself was satisfying. For it refined our oversimplified views of the problems of obese people. The more I learned about the subject, the more I came to realize the importance of being as specific as possible in relating neurosis and obesity. Many obese people have severe neurotic problems. It has all too often been inferred from this fact that the neurosis is a cause of the obesity—and this inference is quite unjustified.

The examination of adult-onset obese people revealed some who were severely neurotic, but whose neurosis did not explain (nor was it even relevant to) their obesity. They could undergo severe mid-life depressions, in response to business reverses or family turmoil, without in any way becoming concerned about their obesity, or even showing any change in their eating patterns or body weight. Any understanding of the relationship of neurosis to obesity requires careful description of which neurotic features are specific to obesity and which are not. The disturbance in body image is one such specific feature.

There is strong evidence that the disturbances in body image of obese people have their origins during a relatively short period of time—when emotionally disturbed adolescents incorporate the derogatory views of peers and parents into enduring views of the self.

We do not have to look far for the frustrations of obese adolescents. Almost all report heart-breaking accounts of the pervasive ridicule to which they have been subjected. Indeed the pattern of discrimination against obese adolescents is so intense and far-reaching, that they could well qualify as a (heretofore unrecognized) minority group.

A brilliant series of recently conducted studies of fat tissue have helped to explain the remarkable persistence of childhood-onset obesity and the special characteristics of people suffering from this condition. These studies have shown that animals and people with childhood-onset obesity have a greater number of cells in their fat tissue than do those with adult-onset obesity. Over-feeding in early life results in both an increase in cell size *and* in total number of fat cells. When an animal is made obese in adult life, on the other hand, he grows no new fat cells; the ones he has simply enlarge.

An adult with juvenile-onset obesity may have five times as many fat cells as one whose obesity began in adult life. With weight reduction, individual cells shrink greatly, but the total number of cells remains constant. The special character of the fat tissue of childhood-onset obese people sets them apart biologically from their adult-onset counterparts. And the special character of this fat tissue may well mean that reducing to so-called "ideal weight" by adult-onset and childhood-onset obese people have quite different consequences. The fat cells of the adult onset obese may simply be reduced to a normal size, while the far more numerous fat cells of the childhood-onset obese are being severely depleted of their fat stores.

The more I have thought about the implications of this work, and reviewed my experience with childhood-onset obese people, the more I have wondered whether at least some degree of overweight on the part of these people may not be normal for them. They can achieve weight loss to statistically "normal" levels—but perhaps only at the cost of living in a state of semi-starvation. Small wonder that they have emotional problems and are vulnerable to depression.

seven

Psychotherapy and Obesity

The ultimate concern of physicians—whatever they may do and however far they may stray from it—is treatment. This concern, perhaps more than any other, distinguishes physicians from scientists. Admittedly their interests may converge, and they are frequently dealing with the same issues. But the two approach their work with clearly distinctive goals.

The scientist is ultimately interested in knowledge, and theoretically there is no limit to the extent of his inquiry. In fact the quest of the scientist never stops. Each new discovery gives birth to a new theory, which suggests a new discovery . . . and so on, without end. The eventual aim of the physician, on the other hand, is to make a decision; and the better the physician, the more he seeks to know. But, in distinction to the scientist, there is a point at which his search must stop. Using the information available, he must act on it.

The most important decisions that a physician makes are those about treatment. Thousands of times each day in the United States, physicians reach critical judgments about treatments for obesity. And every year tens of millions of Americans attempt weight reduction.

Of course the doctor's office is no longer the sole province of dieting advice. With enormous fanfare, new schemes for weight reduction are constantly turning up in magazine articles and how-to books. The paths to slenderness seem countless. There are high-protein diets and low-protein diets, high-carbohydrate diets and low-carbohydrate diets, high-fat diets and low-fat diets, rice diets and banana diets, the "drinking man's" diet, and the "prudent" diet, and even (defying the laws of thermodynamics), a diet in which we are told "calories don't count." Fasting has come into considerable vogue, as have appetite suppressants like the amphetamines, and exercise programs of one strenuous sort or another.

Some of these regimens are harmful; others are not. Any given approach may be successful for one person (at least in the short run), but useless or even disastrous for another. Basic to most, however, is the unrealistic notion that there is a cure-all for obesity. We are led to believe that weight loss is a simple matter: it requires only the reduction of caloric input to levels lower than output. And, in the last analysis, that is true. But its very simplicity leads to an illusory sense of ease about the task. It should be easy. But is it? What are the results of medical treatment for obesity?

Repeatedly, we have learned the distressing answer: Most obese patients will not enter medical treatment for obesity; of those who do, most will not lose a significant amount of weight; and of those who do lose weight, most will regain it.

What about psychotherapy? Has it proven any more successful than these other methods? Again, the findings are disheartening. *Obesity is a chronic condition, resistant to treatment and prone to relapse.*

Of course information about reducing diets is so widely available that only people who have already failed to lose weight on their own come to the doctor's office. And only the failures from medical treatment reach the office of the psychiatrist. In this context it is perhaps easy to understand why psychotherapy seems to have been no more effective than other, less expensive, aids to weight reduction. Less understandable is the widespread belief in the effectiveness of psychotherapy. Many people are convinced that it is the only truly definitive treatment for obesity. There is no evidence to support this belief.

It is my belief that psychotherapy *cannot* change the basic pattern of over-eating in response to the stress that is so common among obese people. Years after even successful psychotherapy and successful weight reduction, people who have over-eaten under stress continue to do so.

Does this mean that psychotherapy has no place in the treatment of obesity? Decidedly not. Although in all probability the pattern of over-eating in response to stress cannot be changed, psychotherapy can help obese people live less stressful and more gratifying lives. When this occurs, they are less apt to over-eat. They may even reduce and stay reduced.

The first question to be answered concerning psychotherapy, and one which is all too often left unresolved, is whether it should be undertaken at all. My earlier experience with dieting depressions had driven home the fact that psychotherapy is not necessarily harmless. As is perhaps true of any kind of treatment, the capacity to heal may carry with it the possibility of harm; and the decision to undertake psychotherapy requires careful assessment of the likelihood of each outcome. For even when there is no outright harm, treatment can bog down in a prolonged and painful therapeutic impasse. The patient may receive little or no benefit, and his energies and attention may be diverted from more rewarding activities in the real world. For patients and therapists caught in such impasses, it is often difficult even to recognize the problem, let alone terminate treatment.

The psychotherapist's first step in determining whether treatment should be undertaken is to find out from the patient what he considers his problems to be, his strengths in coping with these problems, and what he hopes to gain from the treatment. In the course of learning about these matters, the psychotherapist also usually learns a great deal more about other matters, of which the patient himself is not fully aware. The critical judgment as to whether to undertake treatment should depend in large measure upon the therapist's assessment of his ability to help the patient achieve reasonable goals, without undue risk and without excessive investment of time and effort.

The importance of an early agreement between patient and therapist upon the goals of therapy cannot be overstated. I expect that psychotherapy has come to grief over a failure to reach such agreement during this initial period, as frequently as from any other problem. Conversely, psychotherapy has often been carried out successfully in the face of forbidding odds, largely because of a clear contract between the patient and the therapist as to what they were proposing to do.

My initial conversation with Herbert Marx left me uncertain as to the degree to which we had achieved, or could achieve, agreement on goals and expectations. Many of the signs were favorable: Herbert's earlier psychotherapy had helped him to think systematically about his problems, and his initial formulation of them was reasoned and thoughtful. All three complaints which he formulated—"inconsistency, unpredictability, and going to extremes"—were clear and disturbing kinds of behavior; and he described them and the associated difficulties articulately and well. Within a short period of time I was able to construct in my own mind a sense of how he viewed himself and his world.

I could even feel his sense of being an indulged and helpless child who had really only one task in the world—to control his eating and his body weight. Success in this task meant continuation of a warm and happy life. And the task seemed, on the face of it, to be a simple one. But to Herbert's distress, mysterious forces always seemed to sweep in upon

him, to overwhelm him and force him to over-eat and gain
weight despite his every effort. The result was estrangement
from everything he held dear, and his descent into a world
of misery and self-hatred.

Because of this pervasive self-derogation I approached
the effort to define our treatment goals with some uneasiness.
But his first definition was reassuring: "I guess I would just
like to feel free and easy—not to feel inferior, not to always
feel like I'm an outsider." I was moved by this honest, human
wish. It seemed like a realistic goal, and one which I expected
he would work hard to achieve. I felt the same way about
his more specific goal: dating Gladys. Beyond that, I liked
Herbert from the first. And, as recent research has shown,
the therapist's liking for his patient is as important to the
outcome of treatment as are his positive expectations. Both
are predictive of success.

Another important predictive factor is the degree to
which the patient can relate his symptoms and his disturbed
behavior to specific problems in his life. Since a great deal
of psychotherapy involves discovering just such relationships,
evidence that the patient has some native ability bodes well
for the outcome of treatment. If, on the other hand, the patient
comes to treatment with no apparent ability to see connections
between his problems and his symptoms, he isn't likely to
develop it during treatment. To some degree every neurotic
person has failed to make such connections, and Herbert Marx
was no exception. His description of the way in which the
impulse to eat would arise out of the blue and suddenly
overwhelm him conveyed his mystification as to what was
happening to him. I had the sense, however, that down deep
he had at least a rudimentary understanding of his difficulties.
He showed no hesitancy in relating his "loss of ambition to
date" to his mother's unfavorable response to his date with
Gladys. And he spoke with some insight into the origins of
"the terrible summer" when his weight had risen from 160
to 260 pounds.

But, beyond these proofs of awareness, there was another
element that influenced my assessment. In trying to predict

the prospects for a patient entering psychotherapy, I have generally placed a good deal of importance on certain kinds of incidents, incidents which show that the patient's symptoms or disturbed behavior can be interrupted by some kind of human contact. At the time of his second visit, Herbert reported one such episode which moved me deeply and gave me greater hope for his treatment than I otherwise might have had. Each of us referred to it at times, and it became a source of comfort to us both during dark periods.

About the time Herbert had started treatment, he was accepted into the graduate program of a local institute of technology. But this good fortune had had no effect upon his misery or his over-eating, and he had dismissed it with a shrug when I complimented him about it. Then, the day after his second visit to me, he over-ate during the morning, and ". . . I decided to really go out and ruin the day. I was just leaving Mother's house to go down to the bakery to get some food and start bolting it down when I met Ruth. She's a neighbor of my mother's, and she's a freshman at Drexel. When she saw me, she came right up and congratulated me on getting accepted into the graduate course, and then she welcomed me into the Drexel community.

"What happened next was really amazing. By the time I got in the car I'd decided against starting on a binge, and so I drove on down the street and past the bakery. I had the thought, 'It's not too late. You still have friends!' My optimism started to return. So I drove on to the drugstore and bought a roll of film instead."

I asked Herbert if anything like this had ever happened before, and he said he thought so, but rarely. "I hardly ever see girls at all any more. I feel even more inferior around girls than I do around boys. But then I felt, 'Well, at least one girl accepts me.' And it didn't take more than a minute to call off the binge."

I remember marveling at the time about how one of Herbert's voracious eating binges could be aborted by such a small human event. It gave me hope. I felt that if such a small show of human kindness could interrupt his agony so decisively, somehow I would have to help him to become better acquainted with this sort of experience.

Once having decided that the prospects of success in psychotherapy are sufficiently high, and the probability of injury to the patient sufficiently low, what do we do when we undertake psychotherapy? What is it that happens in the process?

Ever since I read Jerome Frank's insightful volume, *Persuasion and Healing*, I have been influenced by its thesis that psychotherapy consists of two distinct and clearly separable elements. One, "persuasion," consists of learning new forms of behavior and new outlooks on life which are more adaptive to the situation in which the individual finds himself, and more useful in coping with its stresses. "Healing," on the other hand, consists primarily of an increase in feelings of well-being and self-esteem, along with decreases in unpleasant emotions, particularly anxiety and depression.* Whereas persuasion usually requires a certain minimum exposure to the therapeutic process, healing may occur within one visit; and, in fact, it is unlikely to occur at all if it does not begin promptly. Whereas persuasion exerts its effect largely through its influence upon our reason, healing contains a sizable component of irrational elements. Both processes depend to some degree on the skill of the therapist, but healing seems a far more capricious event, and more contingent upon the personal qualities of the therapist.

What goes on in psychotherapy? There must be as many conceptual schemes elucidating psychotherapy as there are therapists, and it is difficult to find a basis for choosing among them. One which appeals to me sees psychotherapy as a

---

*The phenomenon of healing is particularly well exemplified in the so-called "placebo" response. A placebo (from the Latin, "I will please") is a biologically inactive substance, which, when administered to a patient, relieves his symptoms. The effectiveness of placebos in the relief of all manner of symptoms, some physical as well as psychological, has been known for centuries. Indeed, until the advent of biologically effective medicines during the past half century, the history of medicine was very largely one of the placebo effect.

composite of five processes or operations: (1) the use of a special kind of personal relationship to (2) discern the problems, and the strengths, of the patient, to (3) isolate the various elements of the problems, and to (4) devise strategies for coping with these elements and helping the patient implement these strategies, with success leading to (5) increased mastery, especially in personal relationships, with an associated elevation in self-esteem and decrease in painful emotions. This scheme helps to describe what occurred during the treatment of Herbert Marx.

As discussed earlier, the first three months of treatment were spent in a "honeymoon" phase. This period of heightened mood and lessened anxiety is common in all forms of psychotherapy, and is very gratifying to both patient and therapist. Of the two elements of psychotherapy, persuasion and healing, the honeymoon consists largely of healing. Like healing in general, it is poorly understood. In any event, obese people seem no more likely to experience a honeymoon phase of treatment than do the non-obese. Factors other than obesity determine the intensity of the honeymoon and, in fact, whether it occurs at all. Loneliness, for example, must be a powerful stimulus. Desperation, feelings of helplessness, and a sense of personal ineffectiveness all have comparable effects.

Given the predisposition of a patient to experience a honeymoon, what other elements are needed? A critical ingredient, perhaps *the* critical ingredient, is the evocation of hope. It seems to be always present in honeymoons, and absent when a honeymoon does not occur. Patients frequently comment that the early evocation of hope springs from a sense that order is being brought out of the chaos of their lives. Previously inexplicable and depressing reactions of their own and of other people become understandable. They find themselves able to cope with problems which had formerly overwhelmed them.

Such was the honeymoon phase of Herbert Marx's treatment. His first formulation of his problem, in terms of inconsistency, unpredictability, and going to extremes, started the process. There seemed no doubt that the unpredictability of his responses, particularly his eating binges, was a major factor in his profound sense of helplessness. By defining unpredictability as a problem, he narrowed the distressingly large and variable field of painful events to one general class. And he thereby helped to define the nature of our therapeutic task.

One of the major contributions to bringing order out of chaos was to review with Herbert the circumstances of his family life. Prior to these discussions he had been strongly inclined to attribute his unhappiness solely to his inability to control his eating. He seemed quite unaware that the kind of assault which had driven his father out of the family might also have led to his feelings of inadequacy and self-hatred. The notion that his difficulties were not entirely self-inflicted, and that the actions of other people contributed to them, was a source of enormous relief. The discovery that other people could also affect his feelings of well-being, and even play a role in the control of the mysterious and terrifying eating binges, was just as important. For he had exhausted his attempts to regulate his life by controlling his eating, and it was reassuring to learn that his problems lay in his relationships with other people—that they could be dealt with by changing those relationships.

The occurrence of at least a small honeymoon in the form of decreased anxiety and heightened self-esteem is, I think, indicative of future success in treatment. Its occurrence does not insure such success, as was so dramatically demonstrated by the dieting depression. But when a honeymoon fails to develop, treatment is far less likely to be successful.

One of the basic processes of psychotherapy is discerning the patient's problems and also his strengths. The process of discerning Herbert's problems began on the first day of treatment and continued until the last. Often it was unsuccessful, but the discipline of subjecting painful and obscure events to careful scrutiny gradually improved his powers of observation and made him better able to recognize the determinants of his behavior. At times his efforts resulted in greater understanding of painful and confusing events. At times we were able to bring order out of chaos.

The first time we worked out an understanding of a painful and confusing event was during the first period of depression at the end of the honeymoon. What was to become a dominant theme throughout treatment was first uncovered in connection with his giving up his job as waiter at his mother's insistence. The theme was "giving in to her and becoming her little boy." These discoveries first conveyed to Herbert something of the nature of the heretofore obscure forces which had swept through his life, bringing in their wake bleak helplessness and self-contempt.

There was a comparable experience during another period of binging and weight gain. It occurred at the time when Herbert's relationship with Gladys was becoming disturbingly ambiguous. With encouragement he was able to ask her about her feelings towards him. The answer was painful and it ushered in a second period of depression. But the episode was important, for it served as a model for forming and testing a hypothesis about a painful relationship. And it gave him some experience in dealing with such a relationship in a straightforward way.

Straightforward dealings with people had not been Herbert's strong suit. Nowhere was this more apparent than in his relationships with his mother; and over a period of time we examined some of his obscure and devious interactions with her. He learned to his surprise that this behavior had not been his own invention, but rather one he had learned from a skillful teacher.

One such episode stands out. It occurred during Herbert's first period of depression. He had declined an invitation to a Bar Mitzvah because he felt so inferior and believed that attending it would make him too uncomfortable. His mother knew the family which was holding the celebration and had heard about his declining the invitation. She wanted to find out the reason, but apparently could not bring herself to ask him directly. So she did it indirectly, by asking him if he would help her in the store on the day in question. He replied with some indignation, "How can I, Ma? You know I am going to the Bar Mitzvah."

There ensued a long sparring match, and eventually Herbert admitted having declined the invitation. Puzzled, I later pressed him for an explanation of this curious behavior. There was an edge of anger in his voice as he said, "I did it because I wanted to make her squirm. I hate her deviousness."

The discernment of these various problems played an important part in Herbert's growing understanding. But the most important instance of growth during the first year of treatment required no special effort and occurred almost casually. Once the honeymoon phase of treatment had conferred a modicum of comfort, and he dared to hope, he decided, "I'm all set for the next step; now I want to have a date." And no longer setting the arbitrary weight barrier of reaching 160 pounds, he began to plan how to ask Gladys.

In helping him to screw up his courage, I found myself developing a treatment strategy which I have continued to use since then. The strategy consists, quite simply, of encouraging the patient to talk about a specific goal or aspiration. Once the patient begins to talk, I listen attentively, nodding encouragement, and indicating approval—anything to keep him talking about the goal. When he deviates from the topic, I look away, fail to respond, and give no encouragement.

Over the weeks I discovered that judicious application of attention could cause Herbert's talk about dating to move in ever more specific channels. First it was the rewards which he expected to gain from dating, then statements of confidence in his ability to overcome his fears, then more and more concrete plans, leading up to the idea of writing Gladys. And then finally came the day when he came into the office to announce that he had actually written to her. His exuberance was touching; and her prompt and friendly reply fully rewarded his initiative.

In encouraging Herbert to see Gladys these tactics seemed to work even more dramatically. Very small instances of attention were sufficient to keep him talking about dating her. And even when this conversation began with an account of his fears of meeting her, he would soon shift to more resolute statements and more hopeful fantasies. In less than a month his confidence about being able to see Gladys rose sharply, even though he had not yet seen her. I had only just begun to wonder whether he would continue to talk so bravely in the interviews and fail to act, when he told me that he had finally seen her. Again, the strategy seemed to have worked.

But the triumph was short-lived. When Gladys eventually rejected Herbert for another man, I discovered that my ability to modify the content of his talk almost disappeared. For whatever reason, and probably because my tactics were no longer rewarding to him in his depressed state, I found myself unable to interrupt the recurrence of his interminable ruminations about his eating, his body, and his despair.

Herbert's depression finally subsided, at the same time that he increased his ability to cope with his family. His interest in dating revived, and in these altered circumstances his responsiveness to my rewarding the content of his speech increased dramatically. So I immediately started reinforcing his talk about dating. Within a month he entered the office, radiating confidence, to announce, "I made a certain phone call today." His second experience in dating had begun.

This was the very same day on which he had left his uncle's house, telling his family he would look elsewhere for a place to live. In one fell swoop, Herbert tasted the fruits of success in both his social and his family relationships. It is difficult to say which was the more important in its favorable effect upon his body image. But whatever the cause, the effect was striking. Despite his weight of 240 pounds, Herbert was jubilant. "God knows why, but it's gotten so that I almost *feel* thin . . . I feel that I'm in command now." With these confident words, he entered a new phase of treatment; and we will continue his story from the previous chapter.

I soon had ample opportunity to examine the effects of this new strategy, for Herbert's second experience in dating turned out as unhappily as the first. But this time his reaction was far less intense. After a temporary halt, he returned to the quest with renewed enthusiasm. When one girl turned down his invitation, he simply called another. "I'm trying harder now than I ever did before. I know I'm going to get turned down and have unhappy experiences. But I'm going to keep trying until I get a date."

We reflected upon the difference from the year before, when his desperation had led to decreased activity and depression. Now it was leading to action. He no longer felt helpless. He was developing a sense of mastery about dating, and this was sufficient to make him feel optimistic. Systematically, he went about trying to get a date, with no special emotion and with low expectation of success. Over the weeks his effectiveness increased and his efforts paid off. Girls began to accept his invitations. But their acceptance was less important than it would have been formerly. "Just my asking them out is the important thing. It doesn't really matter so much whether I have a date or not as long as I can ask a girl for one."

This increased self-confidence spread into other areas of his life. "Today some nurses got in the elevator after I got on to come up to your office. This used to frighten me so much that I used to get out when they got in. I just felt that they would have complete disgust for me, total revulsion, because I was so fat. Today it didn't bother me at all. Now I'm thinking like a person of normal weight. I just think I'm doing the best I can. Not in respect to weight, of course, but in living the best way I can, not staying up too late at night, getting up in the morning on time, and when I study, studying the important things first and leaving the others till later, or even not doing them at all. No great fireworks, but it feels good."

Herbert found, when he began to date at the age of 23, that he really didn't know much about it. He had missed the typical experiences of his age group, and his naiveté resulted in some blunders. Once, for example, he decided to follow the advice of a classmate to "diversify"—to date different girls. But his diversification consisted of trying to date the best friend of a girl he was then dating.

But he continued to try and to learn from his efforts. And his experiences modulated the unrealistic fantasies he had dreamed during the years of loneliness. "I used to believe that people on dates are the most wonderful people in the world. Now I'm finding that they are just people after all, and dating is just like a lot of other things in life."

His increasingly realistic appraisal of dating and his determination to succeed at it made the process easier and easier. "It's almost like an adventure. I keep looking forward to seeing how things will turn out." Even disappointments could no longer set him back. For example, on one occasion he was turned down for a date by a girl he had come to like. "When I hung up the phone I felt crushed and terribly angry at her. I felt 'Goddamn women . . . who needs them anyway?' Then that evening I had a dream. I really can't remember the details. All I know is that I asked her to go out and she said yes." Herbert went on talking about the girl and his anger and how he felt: "I'll never ask you out again, sister. The hell with you. We're through." Then, as we talked further, he realized that he wanted very much to go out with her again and that his dream had been a simple fulfillment of this wish. He took a deep breath, sighed and smiled. Then he left the office and called her again.

Let me backtrack at this point to an earlier stage of Herbert's therapy in order to consider another aspect of treatment: helping the patient to discern his problems. Eating binges provided a good opportunity, for I had had considerable experience with them, and Herbert Marx had quite typical binges. He described their occurrence, as I had come to expect, as "sudden . . . unpredictable . . . out of the blue." He told of how they frightened him by showing the extent to which his life was controlled by irrational forces. I was able to tell him that my experience with other patients made me confident that his binges had quite specific causes. What is more, I told him, I believed that systematic, disciplined study of his binges would enable us to discover those causes. I told him that eventually I thought that he would be able to control the causes and, thus, the binges.

He took heart from this formulation and began paying attention to what preceded his binges. For a long time, his effort bore little fruit. During the honeymoon phase of treatment he had few binges. Then, when he became depressed, he felt too discouraged, particularly after a binge, to review in a disciplined manner what had preceded it. His efforts produced either detailed lists of minutiae or very general statements about feeling angry, bored, or frustrated.

Eventually, however, our low-keyed but insistent inquiry increased his awareness of events which preceded his binges. Nearly a year after treatment had begun, he said that he had been mulling over this matter and the anger which was usually present. "But there's something more than anger." He paused, frowned, and said slowly, "It's a feeling that someone is imposing their will on me."

Then Herbert had a binge which confirmed this supposition. It occurred during the period of exhiliration that had followed his first date with Gladys. A good part of this joy had stemmed from what he saw as Gladys' acceptance of him as a man—and one aspect of manhood, as he saw it, was the kind of clothes you wore. For years he had envied men who dressed in the Ivy League style which he had seen in the windows of men's stores. And for years he had let his uncle buy his clothes for him at the cut-rate, wholesale clothing store which belonged to a distant relative of the family.

Now, in the full flush of his newly-won manhood, he announced that he was going to buy himself an Ivy League suit at a men's store. The scene of this announcement was his aunt's house, and her righteous reaction stunned him: "Don't you go getting any ideas about buying clothes by yourself . . . And stay away from men's stores. If a men's store ever got its hands on a soft touch like you, they'd rob you blind."

He continued morosely, "It was just more of the same attitude that they've always had about me. I'm all right as a person who can memorize from books, but I don't know anything about the real world.

"Then my cousin said that if I really needed a new suit so badly she would go out and buy one for me. Then my aunt got into the act and said no, that my cousin wasn't going to buy any suit for me. There was no reason why my uncle shouldn't take me down to the wholesale dealer's like he'd always done, and that he knew good material when he saw it and wouldn't be cheated. It was like they were taking over . . . They seemed so positive."

For just a few moments Herbert had been angry, and then he began to back down. Their ideas seemed right. He began to wonder how he had ever thought that he would be able to buy a suit by himself. It somehow just seemed like the right thing for him to go down to the wholesale store with his uncle. "Then I noticed that I had this overwhelming desire to eat. So I left the house and went to a store around the corner and had myself an enormous binge."

As we continued to study Herbert's binges, we became able to distinguish their different elements. Frequently they were preceded by an interaction with someone who, as Herbert put it, "tried to impose his will on me." If he gave in, there was usually a period of tense anticipation. Thoughts of food would arise and become increasingly intense. Then came the binge, with all of its sequelae. Gradually we began to recognize that the critical time in this sequence was the period of discomfort between the precipitating circumstances and the actual eating. At first Herbert was quite unaware of any such period. Then, when he finally became aware of it, it was rarely more than four or five minutes before he found himself compelled to eat. As we continued to study individual binges, this interval increased, to an hour, or even two. When the interval became this long, we could begin to devise strategies for aborting the binge.

It seemed as if Herbert was experiencing intense, if sometimes poorly perceived, anxiety during this latent period. We therefore explored the possibility of his taking some medication during this critical time. With some misgivings, he began to carry in his pocket one or two tablets of a minor tranquilizer. When he thought that a binge was threatening, he was to take them. For some time this strategy didn't work at all. He could never be completely sure that a binge was actually impending, and he felt that it would be improper, even immoral, to take a tranquilizer unless he could be certain that he was about to have a binge. For a time only the onset of a binge could give him this certainty, and by then it was too late. Eventually, however, he became able to take the medication, even when he was in doubt about the imminence of a binge.

Not unexpectedly, this new attitude ushered in a period of fewer binges. We never knew for sure whether this favorable development was due to the pharmacological effects of the medication. Certainly the fact of doing something on his own behalf during critical situations made him feel less helpless and gave him a sense of mastery over situations which had formerly filled him with dread. From this time on he became increasingly able to use the occurrence of a binge to examine, and often to correct, what was going wrong in his life.

The next step was to help Herbert come to grips with his relationship with his mother. Hoping to increase his aware-ness of it, I resorted again to the technique of influencing the content of his talk. Whenever he told me of something his mother had said, I showed special interest and encouraged him to continue. Soon he was recounting the long, detailed, emotion-ridden descriptions of his dealings with his mother. As he became progressively caught up in these descriptions, he started asking his mother more and more about her feelings regarding obesity. In this active role, he became able to toler-ate her vicious attacks upon obesity and obese people. The helpless, frightened boy who could deal with his mother only in devious and obscure ways gradually became an assured and careful investigator.

As Herbert continued to report ever more outrageous sentiments on the part of his mother, I detected a shift in his attitudes towards her. Initially he had seemed frightened as he described his mother's assaults; then he seemed awed. Soon I began to hear a note of incredulity, and, finally, anger. Carefully assessing the quality of his emotion, I made every effort to reward him for statements which showed evidences of assertiveness.

It was at this time that Herb received the note from his mother saying that he was a terrible disappointment to

the people who loved him, and asking why he did not appreciate their love. This had aroused the first overt expression of
anger towards her. He had slammed the letter upon my desk
and snarled, "What the hell does she think she's doing, sending
me letters like this?"

From this point on it was relatively easy to encourage
similar statements and feelings. Soon afterwards, while describing how his aunts disparaged him, he made his intense
vow, "I'll never allow them to do this to me again." And
only two weeks later he took on his uncle, the first clear-cut
expression of anger towards a family member that he could
remember. Soon he found himself arguing, angrily and effectively, with his aunts.

It was several months before Herbert's new-found ability
to struggle with members of his family extended to his mother.
A typical interchange between the two helps illuminate this
difficulty. It occurred regularly during the telephone calls
which he made every evening at her request. She would begin
the conversation with an account of her troubles and of how
much she had suffered during the day. "After a while I get
to feeling very sympathetic toward her. I get so that I want
desperately to help her. I feel that I would do anything to
help her because she is suffering so much. Then, just when
I can hardly stand it any more, she tells me that it's all my
fault because I am a pig and I eat so much. She keeps getting
angrier and angrier as she talks about it and I get all mixed
up. I feel that if my mother is angry, I'm so attached to her
that I have to be angry too. But there is no one to be angry
at except myself . . . By the time I hang up I'm feeling just
terrible."

This kind of episode occurred so regularly and so consistently that I felt it must have deep roots. Herbert confirmed
the speculation: "I remember once when I was little and
Mother's Day was coming up. I knew how much Mother
wanted to be loved, and I wanted to show her how much
I loved her, so I went to my aunt and she helped me to get
Mother a present. I wrapped it up for her and wrote a card
telling her how much I loved her. Then Mother's Day came,

and Mother wouldn't even accept the present. She said, 'No, no, I can't accept presents from my children because they don't love me.' "

As we continued to explore Herbert's relationship with his mother, we became aware of an entirely new element in his perception of her. He still saw her as a fierce, powerful person who could overwhelm him despite his best intentions. But now, side by side with this image, another began to appear, an image of a dangerously frail and vulnerable woman. It was an image which had been painted in large part by his aunts. From his earliest years he could remember them enjoining, "Don't get Mother upset!" He was never sure exactly why it was so important that Mother should not be upset, but he had a sense that there would be terrible repercussions.

"I thought maybe she would get sick, or that she would get so upset that she would insult the customers and we would lose the store and all our money. She's always talking about how sick she is. I'm afraid that if she gets upset this will make her even sicker." He paused and then went on, frowning, "I guess I really feel that if I make her angry it will kill her. I just can't take any chances on upsetting Mother." Again he paused. He shook his head as if incredulous over what he was about to say: ". . . *And if you upset Mother, you upset the balance of the world!*"

Discovering how vulnerable Herbert felt his mother to be took several months, and we spent several more discussing and clarifying his feelings about her. Gradually he relaxed the constraints against telling her how he felt. Two and a half years after he began treatment, he finally felt free enough to bring the quarrel into the open. The first round was a disaster.

He decided to do battle during the evening telephone call. He girded himself for her assault and prepared some choice remarks for replies. He waited until eleven o'clock at night in order to make sure she was alone. ". . . And when I reached her, she was still downstairs, working in the store. I just felt terrible about what I was planning to do. I really was ashamed of myself. I just couldn't go through with it."

If this evidence of his mother's back-breaking schedule aroused Herbert's guilt, she soon provided fuel for other feelings. ". . . I didn't call her yesterday so she called me. And she was just like a mad woman, hysterical and angry and striking out in all directions. She called me a pig. She said that I was so ugly and fat that of course girls didn't want to go out with me. She said that I might as well give up trying. She said she couldn't imagine a girl who would let me touch her."

Herbert went on. "Mother feels that my very being is loathsome." I agreed that this might be true, and reminded him that until a year or so ago he had felt the same way. Even now, occasionally, when he felt badly, these feelings would come back. We discussed why this should be so.

The viciousness of his mother's attacks could quite reasonably be interpreted as her unconditional rejection of him. But this interpretation frightened him. He had preferred to believe that her rejection was a conditional one, that he was being rejected, that is, because he was fat. This left some grounds for hope, for it implied that if he could only lose weight, then his mother would love him. "The thought that she might really hate me is just too terrible to imagine. So if she says that I'm a shit, I go out and prove that she's right by over-eating. My only hope is that the fault is in me and that I can change. If the fault is in her, then there's nothing to be done about it." Abruptly Herbert stopped. When he finally began again, it was with an expression almost of disbelief: "You know, all of a sudden I've gotten a terrible need to eat."

We continued another year. One by one we considered the obstacles to direct confrontation with his mother, and then resolved them. He later said that a major step in his emancipation from his mother was learning that she did not love him the way she said she did. When he had first heard of this notion, he said that it had been simply unbelievable. His aunts, and his mother herself, had told him so often how much she loved him that it had become an article of faith.

After all, there were the incredible hours she worked in that miserable store simply to take care of him, put him through college, make him happy. "She was working so hard for me that I thought of her as a kind of god. I always felt that she was so loving that I didn't dare disagree with her about anything. I felt that I would be killing her if I disagreed."

Once Herbert was able to entertain the idea that his mother's love had its limits, things began to move. He grew to understand her harsh and humiliating comments for what they were. First he recognized her hostility; then he came to terms with it. Gradually he realized that he could not change his mother's view of him, even if he were to lose weight. Finally, he was able to cease the quest of winning her over, of making her happy by meeting her impossible terms. And he could go his own way.

Again and again in our interviews he rehearsed a new assertiveness towards his mother, speaking in angry terms of his plans to confront her. When the confrontation finally came, it was almost an anti-climax. After an active Sunday afternoon with friends, Herbert had stopped at the store for a brief visit. As was usual now, he was alert and prepared for trouble. Things went well until just before he left. Then, as he was walking out the door, his mother called after him, "Goodbye, stinker."

He raced back into the store ready for combat. Coldly he asked his mother what she meant by calling him "stinker." Then ensued a real-life version of the fantasied arguments he had enacted so often in my office and elsewhere. Even the presence of his aunt and a number of customers had not stopped him.

His mother met his unexpected outburst with a counterattack, demanding to know, "Do you love me or do you hate me?" Herbert replied that he had mixed feelings about her. To his delight his mother had replied, "No, you can't have mixed feelings. I'm the only one who can have mixed feelings." His mother went on to tell him of all that she had done for him and all that she had given him. He replied that he thought all of her gifts were simply ways of trying to enslave him. "I met every attack head on and I never lost my head. I won."

This battle with his mother marked the end of an era for Herbert Marx. From that point on, his activities took on a new ease and assurance. More and more he was master of his fate. Indeed, mastery became a prominent theme during his fifth, and last, year of treatment. It extended increasingly over his dieting, his dating, and his relations with his family, as well as his feelings about his work. He had always been a good student, but his work had never brought him the gratification it should have. Now, as he realized the fruits of his hard-won achievements in other areas, he came to appreciate his long-standing academic competence.

Herbert increasingly felt a sense of triumph. His growing mastery of his interpersonal problems had a profound effect upon both his disturbance in body image and his eating binges. The disturbance in body image essentially disappeared. The positive effects on his eating binges were not quite so potent. The binges became less frequent and less severe, but they never completely disappeared. Any one of a number of stresses, if he responded passively and with what he saw as self-betrayal, could precipitate an eating binge. It was usually a small one, however, and there was an encouraging aspect to it—its self-correcting nature. For the occurrence of even a small binge became a stimulus for Herbert to begin a careful analysis of the circumstances which had precipitated it; and the results of this analysis would move him towards more appropriate responses to the stress.

Once started, Herbert's competence in his relations with his family increased rapidly. He no longer permitted angry complaints about himself or his characteristics. He asserted himself earlier and earlier in the course of impending trouble. When he had gained some experience in the exercise of his anger in the family, he modulated it. It became easier and easier to achieve his ends by firm and decisive action; anger was less and less often necessary.

He even learned to cope with his mother without having to be angry. "Last time I was home, my cousin was there, and she asked if she could have the vacuum cleaner back, that she had loaned us. Mother told her that I would be glad to take the vacuum cleaner over to her house in my car. It wasn't much, but I decided to do something about it. I told Mother in a very stern voice to speak for herself, and if she wanted me to do something for my cousin to ask me first. One nice thing about it was that my uncle was there and he heard everything. Later, when we were alone, he congratulated me."

Herbert's increased confidence finally manifested itself in weight reduction. After all of the years of failure, this too was almost an anticlimax. Three years after entering treatment he embarked upon a reducing diet, quietly and with no dramatic show of determination. He continued on the diet without significant interruption, losing about ten pounds a month, and reducing from 260 to his target weight of 140 pounds in a year. Even more remarkable, his weight has not exceeded 145 pounds in the ten years and more since then.

His school work, which had always been good, now became excellent. He completed his doctoral requirements in the minimum time and obtained a promising job in industry. Dating was successful and easy. Once he acquired the ability to date, he pursued it enthusiastically, as if to make up for the lost years. For more than a year he "played the field," dating a number of girls. Then one day, three and a half years after he had entered treatment, Herb came into the office and said that the last weekend had been the best one he'd ever had. He had had two dates, but the one on Saturday night had been special. "I liked her and she liked me, and I guess that that's the first time that this has ever happened. When I got back from the date, I told my roommate, 'I've met the girl I'm going to marry.'"

After all of the difficulties Herbert had had in accomplishing so much smaller ends, his courtship of Carol was remarkably easy. They were married the following spring. He continued to see me once a week during the first year of his marriage, and I think that both of us were surprised at how smoothly he adjusted to it. When problems did arise, they were generally of a kind which we had dealt with many times before, in far more aggravated form. His disciplined introspection could usually detect their origins and devise strategies to cope with them with little help from me. It was heartwarming to watch the flowering of this fine young man after all of the painful years.

Soon after his engagement, Herbert happened to meet Jerome, his old college roommate. Jerome was lonely and unhappy, ". . . So Carol got a date for him and we're taking them skating with us this evening." He went on to explain, "I'm in love now, and when you're in love you feel so good that you want to help make other people feel good too."

On Valentine's Day, he told me proudly that he had sent valentines to every member of his family. It was the first time he had ever done this, the first time he had ever even had any inclination to do it. And it gave him a warm feeling as he thought about it. Remembering his unhappy Mother's Day years before, I shared that warmth.

During his first year of marriage, Herbert was given the opportunity of transferring to the West Coast branch of his company, with a major increase in pay and responsibility. Neither he nor Carol had ever lived outside Philadelphia, and for a time they discussed what it would mean to leave their families and friends. Then they decided to go out and look at the job. The visit was a successful one, and shortly after their return, they decided to move to the Coast.

Herbert told me about this decision and how, the evening that they made it, "I was wearing my Ivy League suit, and I went to the mirror in the bathroom and I looked at myself. Then I said, 'You're O.K., fellow. You may not be the smartest guy in the world, or the wittiest or the handsomest, but you're O.K.' "

He paused for a time, reminiscing, and then went on, "I thought about how different it used to be when I looked in the mirror, and how as soon as I looked, I would despise myself and say, 'You shit-head, you putz, you jerk.' I've come a long way since then . . ."

At our last meeting, Herbert spoke about the fight he

had had with Carol's mother over their move. He had had a binge afterwards, but it hadn't discouraged him. We spent this last visit exploring the ways in which he had failed to assert himself with Carol's mother. He knew what he wanted to do; and he was sure that next time he would do it better.

Then our time was up. I had tears in my eyes when we said goodbye.

Since his move, I have seen Herbert only occasionally, and most of what I know about him is from letters which he sends me at Christmas. Three years after he left, he enclosed a snapshot "of our little pride and joy. She is a happy baby, but she is not nearly as happy as her parents are."

Last year he said simply, "We hope you are well. This has been a year of blessing for us: a new house, a new job (Chief of Section of my Division), and two children who make for hours of work and moments of sheer delight."

eight
Behavior Therapy

The treatment of Herbert Marx had been a long and profoundly moving experience for me. It also marked the end of my efforts to understand obesity through the long-term intensive study of individual patients.

He, and others like him, had taught me a decisive lesson. Psychotherapy could help obese people. Given enough time and effort it could relieve their disturbances in body image and help them control their eating binges. It could even help them lose weight and keep it off.

But this treatment had also taught me another lesson: we would have to look elsewhere to find economically justifiable means for controlling obesity. Individual psychotherapy is time-consuming and expensive. For too many patients, it is a hopelessly extravagant luxury.

But what are the alternatives? If individual therapy is impractical for the great mass of people suffering from obesity, where do we go from here? I have always believed that one day basic biochemical research will provide definitive means of managing obesity. But that could be a long way off, and what do we do until the biochemist arrives?

Happily, further progress has been made, beginning rather unexpectedly. One day on morning rounds, a resident in our Psychiatric Service gave a report on a patient with anorexia nervosa, the curious self-starvation of adolescent girls that was discussed earlier. It was an impressive presentation— warm, concerned, and human, with a scholarly review of the medical literature on the topic.

Anorexia nervosa is a very difficult condition to treat. Young women cling to their semi-starved way of life with incredible tenacity. This tenacity could be lessened by tranquilizers, and so we used them; and with large doses the patients usually began to eat more. But it was an uncertain course of treatment, frequently interrupted by obscure circumstances and sudden reversals. Behind it all lay the central irrationality of the illness—a fear of obesity so intense as to override the most powerful pangs of hunger, and ultimately even the hold on life itself.

The frustrations of trying to treat these women led the residents to search for anyone who might have any suggestions for helping. This search led them to the new and rapidly developing field of behavior therapy.

In general terms, behavior therapy consists of a variety of different therapeutic techniques, bound together by the belief that behavior disorders are learned responses, and that modern theories of learning have much to teach us about the acquisition and extinction of these responses.

Learning theories place great emphasis upon the consequence of behavior—what follows doing or not doing a specific thing. These theories propose that its consequences determine whether or not a form of behavior will continue. Refusal to eat, thus, might be maintained by the consequence that the fear of obesity was lessened. And eating, might be restored by following it with a consequent reward that was more powerful than this fear. But what reward could possibly compete with the pervasive anxiety with which these girls had learned to live?

The search for rewards did not at first look promising. One of the striking characteristics of patients with anorexia nervosa is a widespread inhibition against most normal activity. Tense and frozen in appearance, they are a cheerless lot, for whom all pleasure and satisfaction seem to have long-since departed. It was hard on the face of it to think of anything they might find rewarding. Then a related study suggested a possible approach.

We had been using pedometers to investigate the physical activity of anorexia patients, looking into the as yet unsubstantiated belief that they are unusually active. The results began to come in, just when we needed them, clearly demonstrating that physical activity was indeed very important to these patients. Was it important enough to start them eating again? We would soon see. A set of ground rules was established, by which patients could gain access to freedom to exercise by gaining weight.

The first resident to tell his patient about the new rules was met with an explosion of fury, and threats to run away from the hospital. The nurses were subjected to equally angry outbursts, and then pitiful pleading that she be let out of the building for walks, whether or not she gained weight.

Four days after the new program was instituted, this patient's morning weigh-in showed a weight gain of nearly a pound. She stopped complaining, and during the next week gained almost six pounds. This surprising change continued, with weight gains of five pounds a week. And that wasn't all. Her tense, frozen manner thawed; she began to seek out and talk with other patients and nurses. She reported that she felt better, and her voice and manner made it clear that she did.

These results made a very strong impression on me. For years I had known about the difficulties of treating people with anorexia nervosa, and although I had personally treated only a few, I had learned to be satisfied with limited goals and long hospitalizations. Suddenly, here was a disarmingly simple technique and what is more, one which worked. Inevitably, I began to think about its application to the treatment of obesity. If such a simple program could be so effective in a condition as stubborn as anorexia nervosa, why couldn't a similar approach help obese people to lose weight?

It did. There were a number of false starts, but also the encouragement of a report that someone had gotten behavior therapy to work with obese patients. And then it all came together. And it looked as if behavior therapy were more effective than what we had been doing. But was it? We decided to find out.

Our experiment followed the conventional method of comparing the results of treatment of obese people treated with behavior therapy with treatments by traditional methods. But we put behavior therapy to the acid test by loading the dice against it. For the traditional treatment we used almost every method we knew, including medication, dietary counselling, and psychotherapy, and we used two very experienced and effective therapists (a man and a woman) to carry it out. For the behavior therapy, we also selected a man and woman team, but one with no previous experience in behavior therapy. For that matter, they had had very little experience in treatment of any kind.

This contrast in therapists provided a critical test of behavior therapy. If the behavior therapy patients lost more weight than those in traditional treatment, despite the inexperience of their therapists, it would seem that it had to be behavior therapy which made the difference.

Fifteen patients were chosen at random to receive behavior therapy; an equal number received the best "traditional" treatment we could devise. Over a three month period, each group (averaging seven or eight) met weekly for two hours.

The behavioral program had four parts to it: (1) a description of the behavior to be controlled (eating), (2) control of the stimuli that precede eating, (3) techniques to control the act of eating, (4) prompt reinforcement of behaviors that delay or control eating.

Description of the behavior to be controlled. The patients were asked to keep careful records of the food they ate. Each time they ate they wrote down precisely what it was they had eaten, how much was eaten, the time of day, where they were, and how they felt. Most patients have come to share our view that record-keeping may be the single most important part of the program. It vastly increases their awareness of how much they eat, of the speed with which they eat, and the large variety of environmental and psychological situations associated with eating. Despite their years of struggle with the problem, most patients express surprise when they learn from the record-keeping how much they eat and the circumstances surrounding their eating.

Sometimes the record-keeping alone produced surprising results. A middle-aged traveling salesman came to realize for the first time that he over-ate only in his car, which he kept liberally stocked with candy bars, peanuts and potato chips. He thought over the problem, stopped storing food in the car, and promptly lost weight.

Record-keeping helped another patient, a 30-year-old housewife, make a similar discovery: for the first time in her life she realized that anger caused her to over-eat. Having made this discovery she acted upon it. Whenever she found herself getting angry, she would make every effort to leave the kitchen or any place where food was available, and if there were time, she would write down how she felt. She became increasingly able to avoid eating in response to anger, and began to lose weight.

A few weeks of simple record-keeping was sometimes more effective in making people aware of their eating patterns than even long-term intensive psychotherapy. This contrast was particularly dramatic in the case of a Philadelphia matron who had been quite satisfied with her five years of psychotherapy, judged by her psychiatrist to be fairly successful.

"Even though I started psychotherapy because of my

weight, as far as the psychotherapy was concerned I don't
think it proved anything about weight. It just didn't have
anything to do with weight reduction. It made me infinitely
more content with myself. It helped me to live with myself
the way I am. But it didn't have any lasting effect on how
I ate.

"The strongest part of the behavior therapy program was
the realization of what you were eating. My problem—and
I think it's shared by a lot of people—was that I really had
no conception at all of what I ate. When I was in the kitchen,
I would just go from one place to the other and pick up things
and eat them, without any idea of what I ate or even that
I had eaten at all. Keeping those records made me recognize
what I was eating, but writing it down became one terrible
bloody bore. I felt I just had to do it, and so I did, but I
never liked it."

Control of the stimuli that precede eating. The stimuli
which precede eating, and particularly the so-called "discriminative stimuli," play a large part in the eating which follows
them. The concept of a discriminative stimulus comes from
the animal laboratory, where such stimuli as the flashing of
a light or the sounding of a tone may be a signal to an animal
that pressing a lever will produce food pellets or other rewards.
Since the reward never occurs without the discriminative
stimulus, the stimulus is said to "control" the behavior which
is rewarded.

The patients' records showed that their eating occurred
in a wide variety of places and at many different times during
the day. Some noted that if they ate while watching television,
for example, it was not long before watching television made
them eat. It was as though the various times and places had
become discriminative stimuli controlling eating.

In an effort to decrease the number and potency of the
stimuli which controlled their eating, patients were encouraged to confine eating, including snacking, to one place.
So as not to disrupt domestic routines, this place was usually
the kitchen.

A parallel effort was made to develop new discriminative stimuli for eating, and to increase their power. Patients were encouraged, for example, to use distinctive table settings, perhaps a uniquely colored place mat and napkin, with special silver. We made no effort to reduce the amount of food the patients ate, but we did urge them to use the distinctive table setting whenever they ate, even when it was only a between-meals snack.

Several patients carried out these suggestions with great conscientiousness. One diligent housewife, convinced of the importance of this measure, went so far as to take her table setting with her whenever she dined out. She lost weight early and easily. Was it because she had controlled her discriminative stimuli for eating? Perhaps it was; we don't yet know for sure.

Once patients were able to stop pairing their eating with such activities as reading the newspaper and watching television, we encouraged them to make further efforts to make eating a pure experience. They were urged to do whatever they could to make meals a time of comfort and relaxation, and particularly to avoid old arguments and new problems at the dinner table. They were encouraged to savor the food they ate, to make a conscious effort to become aware of it as they were chewing, and to enjoy the act of swallowing and the warmth and fullness in their stomachs.

Development of techniques to control the act of eating. One of the major difficulties in controlling the size of a meal is the fact that no more than a small fraction of the meal is absorbed until at least 20 minutes after it has begun. Solely from the point of view of physical satiation, there is consequently much to recommend a slowing in the rate of eating. Furthermore, such slowing heightens awareness of all the components of the eating process and makes it easier to gain control over them. For these reasons we developed specific techniques to help the patients eat more slowly.

They were urged to count each mouthful of food, or each chew, or each swallow. They were encouraged to practice putting down their eating utensils after every third mouthful, until it had been fully chewed and swallowed. Then longer delays were introduced, starting with one minute towards the end of the meal when it was more easily tolerated, and moving to longer and more frequent delays, and then to ones earlier in the meal.

These techniques and those designed to control the discriminative stimuli produced some enthusiastic testimonials. Among the more enthusiastic were those of Mary O'Brien, a college student whose poise and skillful dressing artfully obscured her 180 pounds. She reported her excitement at the first meeting after Thanksgiving.

"It's the very first time in my life that I can remember getting through Thanksgiving without over-eating, and it was the things we learned here that helped me. I just concentrated on eating slowly, and the first thing I knew the dinner was over and I hadn't had seconds. I even left some of the food on the plate!" She continued this practice, and continued to surprise herself. "A couple of nights ago when I was studying I went into my roommate's room and took a cookie, just *one cookie*, from a box that she had there. I ate it very slowly, chewing it carefully and tasting every part of it. And then I went back to my room to study. I was in absolute awe of myself—was this the same Mary O'Brien who two months ago wouldn't have been able to stop at *ten cookies*, let alone one?—who would have eaten the whole box and then another one if it was there?"

William Schultz, a huge, burly man with a full beard and a hearty laugh, entered the program proclaiming he was a "pessimist." "I've lost weight before—I even lost 80 pounds once—and I've always regained it. I suppose I'll lose weight in this program, but I don't have any confidence at all that I will be able to keep it off."

A month later, shaking his head in disbelief, he reported, "You know, it's amazing. I don't know what's done it. I don't know whether it was slowing down, or concentrating and making it a pure experience or what . . . But when I did these things I really tasted food for the very first time in my life. I *really tasted food!* I can't get over it. When somebody used to ask me if I liked food, I would always say 'Sure I like it.' But I'd never really tasted it before. Before, I could eat half a gallon of ice cream at one sitting and never really taste a single bit of it. Now I eat one spoonful of ice cream and really taste it, and it gives me as much pleasure as a whole half gallon used to."

Prompt reinforcement of behaviors which delay or control eating. Although we devised elaborate systems of reinforcement, I think that the most effective rewards were informal ones, incidental to the structured aspects of the program. Perhaps the most important of these was the great sense of satisfaction which patients developed with their growing exercise of control over eating.

With Herbert Marx still very much on my mind, I remembered how long it had been before patients in more traditional therapy began to talk about feelings of control, and of how important these feelings had been to them. As a result, I was surprised and delighted with the speed with which these feelings began to appear in behavior therapy. In many ways this effect was like the equally unexpected influence of the behavioral program on the anorexia nervosa patients—when their weight gain was matched by a relief from tension and by the development of warmth in their social relations.

As Mary O'Brien explained, "It's like I'm making my own future. I think that what it comes down to is that I've started to take control of my life; it's in my hands now to shape and mold as I see fit. It started with controlling my eating, but now it's much more than my eating. Maybe that's because eating has always meant so much to me."

Mr. Schultz, no longer a pessimist, reported that his wife had asked him if he had increased the number of tranquilizers he was taking because he seemed so calm. "She just couldn't get it through her head that I not only hadn't increased the tranquilizers, I had stopped taking them altogether. I don't know quite why I feel so good, but probably it's because I

feel that I'm calling the shots now. I'm in control. But I sure
as hell don't understand it. It's too easy—it ought to hurt."

One of the major problems of any behavioral program
is how to reward the patient promptly after desired behavior.
Every obese person has had some experience with rewards,
but usually they have been too infrequent and too long de-
layed. As one housewife put it, "Like my husband might offer
to buy me a car if I lost 50 pounds. And I might knock myself
out and lose 30 pounds, which is a lot of weight. But what
did it get me—half a car? I got nothing."

To be effective a reward must be administered promptly
following performance of the behavior it is to modify. Even
a delay until the next weekly meeting is too long. In order
to decrease the interval between the behavior and its reward,
we devised a system which awarded the patient a certain
number of points immediately after each of the activities we
were trying to encourage: record-keeping, counting bites and
swallows, pausing during the meal, eating in one place, and
so on. These effectively provided immediate reward, and as
we gained experience, we added increasingly sophisticated
schedules, such as doubling the number of points earned when
a patient devised and performed an activity which was an
alternative to eating, in the face of strong temptation.

Arrangements with the patients' spouses permitted them
to convert their points into personal rewards: relief from house-
keeping chores, trips to the movies, and money, which they
brought to the next meeting for a donation to the group.
At the beginning of the program the patients decided how
the money should be used. To our surprise they chose very
altruistic courses. Each week the first group donated its savings
to the Salvation Army; the second gave its earnings to a needy
friend of one of the members.

We also devised a system to reward patients for weight
loss, in addition to behavior change. Here we tried to steer
a course between small weight losses which were not a result
of dieting, and weight losses so large that any rewards would
be dishearteningly distant. Patients and their spouses worked
out many of these rewards. Some were conventional, like a

trip to the movies for each five pounds lost, or a new dress for 10 pounds. Others were highly creative. One which became very popular required each patient to buy a pound of suet, cut it into 16 pieces and place them in a plastic bag in a prominent place in the refrigerator. The patient then attempted to visualize this as fat on her body. Every time she lost a pound, she removed one ounce of fat from the bag and tried to imagine its disappearance from her body. If she gained weight, she added an ounce of fat to the bag for each pound gained. When the bag was entirely empty, the group gave her, along with lavish praise, a small prize such as a book or a box of cosmetics.

What were the results of this program? As I mentioned earlier, the proportion of obese patients in the medical literature who lost 20 or more pounds was 25 percent; for losses of 40 or more pounds it was 5 percent. In our control group, treated by conventional methods, the results were very similar: 24 and 0. By contrast, the percent of patients treated by behavior therapy was 53 and 13! The difference was even more striking when judged on the basis of a weight loss of 30 pounds. None of the control patients lost this much; 33 percent of the behavior therapy patients did.

There were two other noteworthy effects of the program. None of the patients dropped out of treatment, in contrast to the strikingly high drop-out rates (from 20 to 80 percent) with conventional treatment. And none of the patients reported ill effects of any kind from the program.

In judging the effectiveness of behavior therapy, these were pertinent considerations. There was another of at least equal importance: how long was the weight loss maintained? It is generally believed that weight lost with reducing diets is rapidly regained; and the few scattered studies on the topic support this viewpoint. But the sad truth is that so few patients have lost any significant amount that the question of maintenance of weight loss has been largely irrelevant. If, however, behavior therapy were to prove a more effective method than those previously available, the question of maintenance would become considerably more relevant. With this in mind, we contacted each of the patients a year after treatment.

The results were surprisingly good. Each of the eight patients who had lost more than 20 pounds had maintained that weight loss; and three of them had lost an additional 20 pounds. Furthermore, one of the patients who had lost 40 pounds during treatment had by this time achieved a weight loss of over 100 pounds.

There was one more intriguing finding. Whereas the patients treated by traditional methods all lost about the same amount of weight, there was great variability in the weight losses of the behavior therapy patients. The five best performers belonged to this group as did the single least effective one, the only patient who actually gained weight during treatment. What does greater variability mean?

No one knows for sure, but the possibilities are intriguing. The weight loss of patients treated by traditional means, which was lower and more constant, suggests the effect of some non-specific factor that is common to all treatment—perhaps the establishment of a therapeutic relationship and the hope which it may evoke. The greater weight loss and its greater variability in the behavior therapy patients suggests that it may be brought about by a more specific factor, one which is particularly effective for certain patients and of little or no help to others. The greater variability thus may imply a greater specificity of behavior therapy.

It has another important implication. If we could predict ahead of time which patients were likely to respond to behavior therapy and which were not, we could concentrate our efforts on the former and increase their chances of success. At the same time we could save the latter patients from one more experience with failure. Unfortunately our attempts at prediction were unsuccessful, as have been those of others before and after us. Our experience with one patient offers a clear example of the difficulty in predicting outcomes.

Joseph Romolo was a 420-pound man in his late twenties, who was referred by the Department of Welfare. He had no job skills, had never held a steady job and had not had any job for years. After a slow start, he learned not only the techniques of behavior therapy but also the ideas which underlay them. (He devised a similar program to help himself stop smoking and followed it successfully.) Much to our surprise, he was one of the two patients who lost more than 40 pounds in the course of treatment. In fact, he was the one who subsequently went on to lose more than 100 pounds. When we last heard from him, he had completed a vocational rehabilitation course and had been at work for over a year. Yet even with the power of hindsight, I don't know now how we could have predicted his success.

This lack of predictability aside, the results of our first trial of behavior therapy were impressive—and not just in terms of weight lost. Even more striking was the increased self-esteem and well-being of those who mastered the technique. But we had to ask, as we had so often before with new treatments for obesity, was this just another fad? To what extent were the effects due merely to the support of the group and our own enthusiasm? How much resulted from the evocation of hope, hope which had so often before led obese people to lose weight and then been followed by disappointment?

The answer was not long in coming. Many research workers have been drawn to this field. The clear description of treatment methods and of the principles underlying them have made it feasible to reproduce treatments with a precision never before possible in research on psychotherapy. Research workers are also attracted by the precision and economy of weight loss as a measure of change. In comparison with the elaborate rating scales necessary to measure changes in anxiety and depression, and the crudeness and unreliability of the results, weight change in pounds is an investigator's dream. Not surprisingly, the past eight years have seen an explosion of research on the behavior therapy of obesity.

In study after study, behavior modification has been systematically compared with a wide variety of alternate treatment methods. And in every instance, those people treated with behavior modification have lost more weight. This kind of unanimity is unprecedented in psychotherapy research.

Given this effectiveness, are there ways that this treatment can be brought to bear upon larger populations? The answer is an emphatic "yes."

The great American love affair with weight reduction has already shown us one way—the patient self-help group. Already 400,000 Americans have joined voluntary non-profit organizations devoted to the control of obesity. But this group is dwarfed by the far larger number of persons who have enrolled in profit-making weight control programs. With three million members enrolled in such programs, private industry has become the largest factor in the effort toward widespread control of obesity in this country.

The next few years may well see a significant increase in the ability to control the critical social influences which affect obese people, as the genius of private industry enlists them in large-scale programs of behavioral control. If this development is coupled, as it probably will be, with further increase in the effectiveness of behavioral methods, we may well witness a phenomenon unprecedented in the history of medicine: management of a major health problem passing out of medical hands and into those of private industry.

These developments are particularly important in light of the major health problems of our time. With the conquest of infectious disease, these remaining problems are largely chronic ones, indissolubly linked to our life styles. Our leading killer, heart disease, which presently accounts for over half of all deaths in America, is a case in point. Except for heredity, every factor known to contribute to heart disease is a matter of personal habit: eating foods high in cholesterol and saturated fatty acids, smoking, inadequate physical activity, insufficient attention to the control of diabetes and high blood pressure, and . . . obesity.

All this can be changed by programs already underway. It is perhaps fitting to end this account on the threshold of these important new developments. I began this research with an attempt to discover something about obesity. Over twenty years later, the exploration continues. We have moved from explanation to action, as we are adding to the old questions of *why* people are obese, new questions of *how* to control obesity. It now appears that a broad scale assault on obesity need not await further biochemical knowledge.

Understanding its social determinants may be enough. The many-sided research on modifying these determinants, already fruitful, gives every promise of continuing productivity.

The problems of obesity are still far from solved. Even the application of our best available technology leaves huge numbers of obese people unhappy and in ill health. But for the first time in many years research already underway gives promise of aid and comfort in the foreseeable future. And this is just the beginning.